Canadian Immunization Guide

Fifth Edition

Fifth Edition — 1998

Published by authority of the
Minister of Health

Health Protection Branch
Laboratory Centre for Disease Control

Également disponible en français sous le titre
Guide canadien d'immunisation

Text prepared by
the National Advisory Committee on Immunization

This Guide was published by the
Canadian Medical Association

© Minister of Public Works and Government Services Canada, 1998
Cat. H49-8/1998E
ISBN 0-660-17444-8

Our mission is to help the people of Canada maintain and improve their health.

Health Canada

Message from the

ASSISTANT DEPUTY MINISTER
HEALTH PROTECTION BRANCH
HEALTH CANADA

All recommendations by the National Advisory Committee on Immunization (NACI) on the use of vaccines in Canada are contained in the *Canadian Immunization Guide*. The Guide will be available on the Laboratory Centre for Disease Control Web site at http://www/hwc/ca/hpb/lcdc. Updates on NACI's new or revised recommendations are published in the *Canada Communicable Disease Report* (CCDR), which is also available on the Web site. Updates can be obtained from the special file in our FAXlink service: you will be able to quickly find the latest recommendations and receive them on your FAX machine. Information on the FAXlink service is included on the inside of the back cover.

A recent readership survey revealed that the Guide ranked as useful or better than other sources of information on immunization. If you have suggestions or comments on this fifth edition, we would be pleased to receive them for consideration for the next edition. You can send your comments to the Advisory Committee Secretariat, Bureau of Infectious Diseases, Laboratory Centre for Disease Control, P.L. 0603E1, Ottawa, Ontario K1A 0L2.

Producing such a publication requires considerable dedication and time on the part of those involved. We would like to thank the National Advisory Committee on Immunization, and the responsible members of the Drugs Directorate and the Laboratory Centre for Disease Control, Health Protection Branch, Health Canada, for producing this Guide.

PREFACE

The fifth edition of the *Canadian Immunization Guide* contains numerous changes from the 1993 version but attempts to remain user friendly. Every chapter has been thoroughly reviewed and updated as needed. New chapters have been added on hepatitis A vaccine, national guidelines for childhood immunization practices, and counselling of those with concerns about immunization.The latter topic is increasingly important as members of the public lose their familiarity with the target illnesses of childhood immunization as a result of the great success of the immunization programs. Illnesses unseen are illnesses unfeared: maintaining parents' commitment to immunization will be an important challenge in the new millennium.

Highlights of some other major changes in the Guide are as follows:

■ Vaccine storage and handling is considered in greater detail, with explicit instructions.

■ Vaccination of immunocompromised hosts is described in more depth.

■ The pertussis chapter is completely revised, with preference stated for acellular vaccines and the list of precautions reduced significantly.

■ The measles chapter now describes the two-dose schedule and omits egg allergy as a contraindication.

■ The poliomyelitis chapter now recommends inactivated vaccine exclusively.

■ The rabies chapter places more emphasis on management of potential bat exposures.

■ The travel vaccine sections have been updated regarding oral cholera vaccine and new typhoid vaccines.

■ Pneumococcal vaccine use is more strongly encouraged; revaccination after 3-5 years is recommended for individuals at highest risk.

Changes in the Guide mirror the extraordinary pace of change in the immunization field. This pace has been challenging for members of the National Advisory Committee on Immunization (NACI), who had to keep producing new statements while revising the Guide itself, a mammoth undertaking. I gratefully acknowledge the hard work and expert contributions of members of NACI, the Immunization Division of the Bureau of Infectious Diseases and other LCDC staff, the Committee to Advise on Tropical Medicine and Travel (CATMAT) and the Advisory Committee on Epidemiology (ACE). Important contributions were made by liaison members from the Canadian Paediatric Society, the Canadian Public Health Association, the Canadian Infectious Disease Society, the College of Family Practice and the Canadian Occupational Health Nurses Association. Close liaison with the U.S. Advisory Committee on Immunization Practices (ACIP) has been invaluable.

David W. Scheifele, MD
Chairman (1994-7)
National Advisory Committee on Immunization

National Advisory Committee on Immunization

Members during 1994-1997
*(*denotes membership in 1998)*

CHAIRMAN

D. Scheifele, MD
Vaccine Evaluation Centre
Vancouver, B.C.
1994-7

MEMBERS

P De Wals, MD *
Université de Sherbrooke
Sherbrooke, Québec
1994-7

B Law, MD *
University of Manitoba
Winnipeg, Manitoba
1994-7

M Naus, MD *
Ontario Ministry of Health
North York, Ontario
1994-7

B Ward, MD *
McGill Centre for Tropical Diseases
Montréal, Québec
1994-7

I Gemmill, MD *
Kingston, Frontenac and Lennox &
  Addington Health Unit
Kingston, Ontario
1996-7

W Schlech III, MD *
Victoria General Hospital
Halifax, Nova Scotia
1996-7

P Orr, MD *
Health Sciences Centre
Winnipeg, Manitoba
1997

G De Serres, MD *
Centre de santé publique de Québec
Beauport, Québec
1997

SA Halperin, MD
Dalhousie University
Halifax, Nova Scotia
1994-7

EL Ford-Jones, MD
Hospital for Sick Children
Toronto, Ontario
1996

Y Robert, MD
Direction de la santé publique
  de la région des Laurentides
St. Jérome, Québec
1994-6

F Aoki, MD
University of Manitoba
Winnipeg, Manitoba
1994-6

P Déry, MD
Centre hospitalier de l'Université Laval
Sainte Foy, Québec
1994-5

S Corber, MD
Ottawa-Carleton Regional Health Unit
Ottawa, Ontario
1994

WL Albritton, MD
University of Alberta
Edmonton, Alberta
1994

EXECUTIVE SECRETARY

J Spika, MD
Bureau of Infectious Diseases
Ottawa, Ontario

ADVISORY COMMITTEE SECRETARIAT OFFICER

N Armstrong
Bureau of Infectious Diseases
Ottawa, Ontario

EX-OFFICIO REPRESENTATIVES

Bureau of Biologics
L Palkonyay, MD *
M Smith, MD
Ottawa, Ontario

Bureau of Infectious Diseases
P Duclos, DVM, PhD *
Ottawa, Ontario

First Nations and Inuit Health
  Programs Directorate
C Mustard, MD
L Bartlett, MD
H Robinson, MD
Ottawa, Ontario

LIAISON REPRESENTATIVES

Advisory Committee on Epidemiology
J Waters, MD *
Edmonton, Alberta

Centers for Disease Control and Preventio
S Hadler, MD
J Livengood, MD *
Atlanta, Georgia

National Defence Medical Centre
R Nowak, Maj
D Carpenter, LCdr
A McCarthy, Maj *
Ottawa, Ontario

College of Family Physicians of Canada
T Freeman, MD *
London, Ontario

Committee to Advise on
  Tropical Medicine & Travel
D MacPherson, MD, Hamilton, Ontario
J R Salzman, MD, Vancouver, B.C. *

Canadian Public Health Association
J Carsley, MD *
Montréal, Québec

Canadian Occupational Health
  Nurses Association
R McLaren RN *
Ottawa, Ontario

Canadian Infectious Disease Society
N MacDonald, MD *
Ottawa, Ontario

Canadian Medical Association
A Carter, MD
Ottawa, Ontario

Canadian Paediatric Society
V Marchessault, MD *
Ottawa, Ontario

Preamble

The National Advisory Committee on Immunization (NACI) provides Health Canada with ongoing and timely medical, scientific, and public health advice relating to immunization. Health Canada acknowledges that the advice and recommendations set out in this publication are based upon the best current available scientific knowledge, and is disseminating this document for information purposes. Persons administering or using the vaccines should also be aware of the contents of the relevant product monographs. Recommendations for use and other information set out herein may differ from that set out in the product monographs of the Canadian licensed manufacturers of the vaccines. Manufacturers have only sought approval of the vaccines and provided evidence as to their safety and efficacy when used in accordance with the product monographs.

TABLE OF CONTENTS

PART 3

PART 4

Part I
GENERAL CONSIDERATIONS

The range of immunizing agents available in Canada continues to expand as new vaccines and immune globulins are licensed, and improvements in or modifications to currently available preparations are made. The use of these agents for both active and passive immunization must, therefore, be evaluated continually as the incidence and significance of the diseases against which they confer protection change spontaneously or as a result of vaccine use. When the incidence of a particular communicable disease falls, the need for continuation of the immunization program concerned must be reappraised and, indeed, may be questioned by the public or health policy makers. There is a danger that successful immunization programs might lead to apathy regarding vaccine use and result in resurgence of the disease unless it can be totally eradicated. Although the ultimate aim of those concerned with immunization is the elimination of vaccine-preventable diseases, eradication is usually a practical possibility only in infections such as smallpox, poliomyelitis and measles, which are restricted to humans and involve no other host.

An ideal vaccine should confer long-lasting, preferably lifelong, protection against the disease with a single or a small number of doses. It should be inexpensive enough for wide-scale use, stable enough to remain potent during shipping and storage, and have no adverse effect on the recipient. Some vaccines come close to meeting these criteria; others do not. Each vaccine has its own characteristics, and generalizations are difficult to make; consequently, each is considered separately in this Guide.

Some vaccines consist of inactivated microbes or purified components. Others, particularly vaccines against viral diseases, contain live microorganisms whose virulence has been attenuated. These have the advantages that the dose is small (minimizing production costs) because the virus replicates within the recipient, and that the stimulus (or process) more closely resembles that associated with natural infection. However, live vaccines demand particular care in many ways: in storage, when they may inadvertently be inactivated; in the choice of the individual immunized, since live agents are usually not appropriate for immunodeficient persons or in some cases for pregnant women; and with regard to changes in virulence and possible spread to contacts of vaccinees and to the environment. Also, because live vaccines produce infection they can on occasion produce some of the symptoms and complications of the disease they are meant to prevent, though at much lower frequency than that associated with the disease.

In this Guide, information is presented on the immunizing agents available in Canada and their use in the prevention of communicable diseases. Recommendations on routine immunization of infants and children are discussed in some detail, and an attempt is made to answer most of the day-to-day queries from providers regarding immunization.

Because of variation among manufacturers' products, precise details on the dosage and route of administration of individual products are not usually given. Readers are referred to manufacturers' labelling and package inserts for this information. As well, the manufacturer has sought approval of the vaccine and provided evidence as to its safety and efficacy only when it is used in accordance with the product monograph. Updates of the information in the product monographs are made infrequently. Recommendations for use and other information set out in the Guide may differ from those set out in the product monograph(s) of the Canadian licensed manufacturer(s) of the vaccine. The advice and recommendations set out in this Guide are based upon the best and most current publicly available scientific knowledge.

Cost-benefit

The World Bank has stated that immunization should be first among the public health initiatives in which governments around the world invest. Vaccination programs are considered to be the most cost-beneficial health intervention and one of the few that systematically demonstrate far more benefits than costs.

Tengs and colleagues reviewed 587 life-saving interventions and their cost-effectiveness and concluded that routine immunization programs for children were among the most cost-effective and among the very few that save more money than they cost (i.e., it costs more not to undertake these programs in terms of lives or life years saved). The cost of the 587 interventions reviewed ranged from less than zero (i.e., those that save more resources than they cost) to more than $99 billion per year of life saved (Table 1). The median cost was US$42,000 per year of life saved.

Many cost-benefit studies of routine immunization programs have been conducted, and they almost always demonstrate a very positive cost-benefit ratio, commonly ranging from 7:1 to 80:1. Very few studies of immunization programs, however, have been or are being conducted in Canada. Recent cost-benefit studies of the introduction of a routine two-dose measles vaccination schedule and of the replacement of the pertussis whole-cell vaccine with the new acellular products have indicated that these two strategies were highly cost-beneficial and in the long term would result in savings of several hundred millions of dollars.

Table 1
Cost per Life Year Saved for Selected
Life-saving Interventions (from Tengs et al)

Measles, mumps and rubella immunization for children	≤ 0
Smoking cessation advice for pregnant women who smoke	≤ 0
Mandatory seat belt law	$69
Mammography for women aged 50	$810
Chlorination of drinking water	$3,100
Smoking cessation advice for people who smoke more than one pack per day	$9,800
Driver and passenger airbags/manual lap belts (vs. airbag for driver only and belts)	$61,000
Smoke detectors in homes	$210,000
Ban on products containing asbestos (vs. 0.2 fibres/cc standard)	$220,000
Low cholesterol diet for men over age 20 and 180 mg/dL	$360,000
Crossing control arm for school buses	$410,000
Radiation emission standard for nuclear power plants	$100,000,000
Chloroform private well emission standard at 48 pulp mills	$99,000,000,000

SELECTED REFERENCES

Division of Immunization, Bureau of Infectious Diseases, LCDC. *Canadian national report on immunization, 1996.* CCDR 1997;23S4:40-1.

Tengs TO, Adams ME, Pliskin JS, Safran DG, Siegel JE, Weinstein MC, Graham JD. *Five hundred life-saving interventions and their cost-effectiveness.* Risk Analysis 1995;15:369-90.

World Bank. *Investing in health.* New York: Oxford University Press, 1993.

General Cautions and Contraindications

A guide to true contraindications to vaccination as well as to conditions considered to be precautions rather than contraindications is provided in Table 2. The table also lists other conditions commonly but inappropriately classified as contraindications, such as mild acute illness with or without fever, mild to moderate local reactions to a previous dose of vaccine, current antimicrobial therapy, and the convalescent phase of an acute illness.

Minor illnesses such as the common cold, with or without fever, frequently occur in young children and are not contraindications to immunization. Such infections do not increase the risk of adverse effects from immunization and do not interfere with immune responses to vaccines. Deferring immunization because of acute mild illnesses often results in incomplete immunization of children who either will need later catch-up vaccinations or will develop vaccine-preventable disease. Moderate to severe illness with or without fever is a reason to defer *routine* immunization with most vaccines. This precaution avoids superimposing adverse effects from the vaccine on the underlying illness or mistakenly identifying a manifestation of the underlying illness as a complication of vaccine use. However, if the vaccine is required because of likely exposure to disease or if the child is unlikely to return to continue immunization in a timely fashion, the vaccine may be given despite the intercurrent illness.

Allergic conditions *per se* (e.g., eczema and asthma) are not contraindications to immunization unless there is a specific allergy to a vaccine component. Special precautions may be required with some vaccines prepared in eggs or avian tissue. The section on egg allergy (page 7) and the sections on individual vaccines should be consulted when dealing with an egg allergic individual. Some vaccines contain preservatives (e.g., thimerosal, a mercurial), trace amounts of antibiotics (e.g., neomycin) or trace amounts of other compounds associated with the production or packaging of the vaccine, to which patients may be hypersensitive. No currently recommended vaccine contains penicillin or its derivatives. Yeast allergy is not a contraindication to immunization unless there has been documented anaphylactic sensitivity to yeast.

There is no evidence to support withholding immunization from anyone for whom it is indicated because of a diagnosis of multiple sclerosis or other conditions considered to involve autoimmunity, or muscular dystrophy. Case-by-case decisions must be made in situations in which the condition is unstable.

4

Table 2
Contraindications and Precautions to Vaccinations

Vaccine*	True contraindications	Precautions†	Not contraindications
All vaccines	Anaphylactic reaction to previous dose of vaccine Anaphylactic reaction to a constituent of a vaccine	Moderate or severe illness with or without fever	Mild to moderate local reactions to previous injection of vaccine Mild acute illness with or without fever Current antimicrobial therapy Convalescent phase of an acute illness Prematurity Recent exposure to infectious disease Personal or family history of allergy
DPT	Anaphylactic reaction to previous dose of vaccine	Hypotonic-hyporesponsive state within 48 hr after prior dose of DPT	Fever ≥ 40.5° C after prior dose of DPT Family history of sudden infant death syndrome Convulsion within 48 hr of prior dose of DPT Family history of convulsions Persistent inconsolable crying lasting ≥ 3 hr within 48 hr after prior dose
IPV	Anaphylactic reaction to neomycin		
MMR	Anaphylactic reaction to previous dose or to neomycin Pregnancy Immunodeficient state	Recent administration of IG (see Table 7)	Tuberculosis or positive TB skin test Simultaneous TB skin testing Current antimicrobial therapy Infection with HIV Egg allergy
Hib			History of Hib disease
Hepatitis B			Pregnancy
Influenza	Anaphylactic reaction to egg ingestion‡		Pregnancy

* DPT = diphtheria, pertussis and tetanus vaccine
  IPV = inactivated poliovirus vaccine, MMR = measles, mumps and rubella vaccine,
  Hib = *Haemophilus influenzae* type b conjugate vaccine.
† The events or conditions listed as precautions are not contraindications but should be carefully considered in determining the benefits and risks of administering a specific vaccine. If the benefits are believed to outweigh the risks (e.g., during an outbreak or foreign travel) the vaccine should be given.
‡ Persons with a history of anaphylaxis or systemic reactions after eating eggs should be vaccinated with influenza vaccine only with caution (see pages 7, 108).

It is prudent to keep vaccinees under observation for immediate reactions or syncope for a period of at least 15 minutes after inoculation or for a longer period if hypersensitivity is a possibility. Epinephrine should be available for immediate use when immunizing agents are injected in order to treat the extremely rare but serious complication of anaphylaxis (see pages 9-13).

Should a significant untoward reaction follow an injection of any vaccine, the provider should postpone further doses, report the reaction to the local public health authority and seek expert advice. The use of fractional doses for continuation of a course of vaccine is not recommended in any circumstances.

Adverse Reactions (see also pages 37-43)

Local or systemic adverse reactions may follow use of immunizing agents. Most are mild and self-limited. Rarely, serious or unexpected adverse reactions may occur. The majority of reactions occur shortly after vaccination, but others may not be manifest for some time. Providers should be aware of the incidence and nature of adverse reactions to immunization agents. Parents and patients should be informed about the benefits and risks of vaccines as well as the risks of the diseases to be prevented. It may be helpful to provide information brochures written in lay language. Signed consent is not required, but **parents or the vaccine recipient must always be provided with the above information and given the opportunity to ask questions. It should be recorded in the patient's record that this has been done**.

Parents and patients should be advised to notify their health care provider about any significant adverse event. To facilitate follow-up of adverse reactions, the lot number and manufacturer of the vaccine should be recorded on the vaccine recipient's medical record. Physicians and other health care personnel should report serious adverse events associated with vaccination to their local medical officer of health. Appendix I contains a list and definitions of events that should be reported. Reporting forms are available from local public health offices. An example of a reporting form can be found in Appendix II as well as in the Compendium of Pharmaceuticals and Specialties (CPS). Local public health offices should forward the reports to the provincial health department, which sends them to the Bureau of Infectious Diseases at the Laboratory Centre for Disease Control, Ottawa. The latter is responsible at the federal level for post-marketing surveillance of adverse events temporally associated with immunizing agents. The Bureau has managed a computerized database on adverse events associated with vaccines administered in Canada since 1987. Confidentiality is constantly maintained. Updated reports on adverse events are published periodically and are available on the LCDC website, and *ad hoc* queries are welcome.

Local reactions usually consist of induration, tenderness and redness at the injection site. More severe reactions, e.g., edema and abscess formation, occasionally occur.

Systemic reactions may include fever, rash, joint or muscle pains, fainting, seizures or other central nervous system symptoms. Fainting immediately after vaccination is usually due to apprehension and should not be confused with anaphylaxis (see page 9).

Allergic reactions, such as urticaria, rhinitis, bronchospasm and anaphylaxis, are rare. They may be due to a specific allergy to any component of the vaccine (which may include antibiotics, egg protein or preservatives). If the specific cause of an allergic reaction following vaccination can be identified, that particular component must **never** be given again. If the specific cause is not identified, no component of the vaccine should be given again except on the advice and under direct supervision of a physician.

Severe reactions, local or systemic, may indicate that additional doses of the same agent should be avoided. The physician should seek expert advice in such an instance.

Anaphylactic Hypersensitivity to Egg and Egg-Related Antigens

Vaccines that contain small quantities of egg protein can cause hypersensitivity reactions in some people with allergies to eggs. The likelihood of such reactions occurring varies considerably among vaccines. Adverse reactions are more likely with vaccines against yellow fever and influenza, which are prepared from viruses grown in embryonated eggs. In contrast, the measles and mumps vaccine viruses most widely used in Canada are grown in chick embryo cell culture (a measles-rubella combination vaccine, Mo-Ru Viraten Berna, contains no avian proteins and can be used without regard to egg allergy). After extensive purification steps, the final vaccine products may contain trace quantities of avian proteins, resembling proteins present in hens' eggs. Anaphylaxis after measles vaccination is rare and has been reported both in individuals with anaphylactic hypersensitivity to eggs and in individuals with no history of egg allergy. In some of these instances, allergy to other components of the vaccine (such as neomycin or gelatin) was hypothesized but not proven.

Because of the concern about rare anaphylactic reactions to measles vaccine, the National Advisory Committee on Immunization (NACI) had previously recommended that skin testing for sensitivity to the combined measles, mumps, rubella (MMR) vaccine be performed in individuals with anaphylactic hypersensitivity to eggs. Recent studies have reported uneventful routine MMR immunization in egg-allergic individuals and in individuals with positive MMR skin tests. Others have reported occasional adverse reactions despite the use of MMR skin testing and graded challenge vaccination. In the largest summary of the literature, none of the 284 children with egg allergy confirmed by blinded food challenge had any problem with routine measles immunization (95% confidence interval 99.0-100%). Routine immunization was tolerated by all 1209 children with a positive egg skin test (95% confidence interval 99.75-100%) and by 1225 (99.84%) of 1227 children with a history of allergy to egg (95% confidence interval 99.41-99.98%).

In view of the cumulative data indicating the safety of measles immunization in individuals with a history of anaphylactic hypersensitivity to hens' eggs and the lack of evidence of the predictive value of MMR skin testing, NACI does not recommend routine MMR skin testing in these individuals. Instead, as with all immunization, NACI recommends immunization by personnel with the capability and facilities to manage vaccine-associated adverse reactions such as anaphylaxis. No special precautions are necessary for children with minor egg hypersensitivity if they can uneventfully ingest small quantities of egg as a food ingredient or if they are immunized with the measles-rubella vaccine that is free of avian proteins. No special measures are necessary for children who have never been fed egg before their MMR immunization, and prior egg ingestion should not be a prerequisite for MMR immunization. The following guidelines should be used for individuals with anaphylactic hypersensitivity to hens' eggs (urticaria, swelling of the mouth and throat, difficulty breathing, or hypotension):

1. Yellow fever vaccine and influenza vaccines that are prepared from viruses grown in embryonated eggs should not be given unless the risk of the disease outweighs the small risk of a systemic hypersensitivity reaction. Re-immunization with yellow fever or influenza vaccine is contraindicated in an individual with a previous anaphylactic reaction to the vaccine.

2. Egg allergy is not a contraindication to immunization with MMR. These individuals may be immunized in the routine manner without prior testing. As an additional precaution, however, it may be prudent to observe them for 30 minutes after immunization for any signs of an allergic reaction.

3. Measles-mumps-rubella vaccine (or measles or measles-rubella vaccine) is contraindicated in individuals with a previous anaphylactic reaction to a vaccine containing one of these components.

4. If there is a compelling reason to re-immunize an individual who has had a prior anaphylactic reaction to the same vaccine, or to administer yellow fever or influenza vaccines prepared in embryonated chicken eggs to an individual with anaphylactic hypersensitivity to hens' eggs, skin testing and graded challenge can be considered. However, because of the possibility of a hypersensitivity reaction to the skin test or during the graded challenge, testing should be performed in an appropriately equipped facility by skilled personnel familiar with the procedures and with the treatment of anaphylaxis.

SELECTED REFERENCES

Freigang B, Jadavji TP, Freigang DW. *Lack of adverse reactions to measles, mumps and rubella vaccine in egg-allergic children.* Ann Allergy 1994;73:486-88.

James JM, Burks SW, Roberson PK et al. *Safe administration of the measles vaccine to children allergic to eggs.* N Engl J Med 1995;332:1262-66.

Anaphylaxis: Initial Management in Non-Hospital Settings

This section is intended as a guide for the initial management of patients in a public health clinic or similar non-hospital setting. In a patient with severe, life-threatening anaphylaxis, establishment of intravenous access for drug and fluid administration will be necessary, and endotracheal intubation and other maneuvers may be required. These interventions are ordinarily best performed in a hospital's emergency department.

Anaphylaxis is a rare and potentially life-threatening allergic complication of vaccination that should be anticipated in every vaccinee. Prevention is the best approach. Prevaccination screening should include questions about possible allergy to any component of the product(s) being considered in order to identify this contraindication. As avoidance is not always possible, every vaccine provider should be familiar with the symptoms of anaphylaxis and be ready to initiate management and administer appropriate medications. Most instances begin within 30 minutes after an injection of vaccine; shorter intervals to onset foretell more severe reactions. Thus vaccine recipients should be kept under supervision for at least 15 minutes after vaccination; 30 minutes is a safer interval when there is a specific concern about possible vaccine allergy. In low risk situations, supervision can include having vaccinees remain within a short distance of the vaccinator (e.g., within a school being used for vaccinations) and return immediately for assessment if they feel unwell.

Anaphylaxis is one of the rarer events reported in the postmarketing surveillance system for vaccine adverse events. Based on the last 5 years of complete national data the annual rate of anaphylaxis ranges from 0.11 to 0.31 reports per 100,000 doses of vaccines distributed.

Anaphylaxis must be distinguished from fainting (vasovagal syncope), anxiety and breath-holding spells, which are more common and benign reactions. During fainting, the individual suddenly becomes pale, loses consciousness and collapses to the ground. Fainting is sometimes accompanied by brief clonic seizure activity (i.e., rhythmic jerking of the limbs), but this generally requires no specific treatment or investigation. Fainting is managed simply by placing the patient in a recumbent position. Recovery of consciousness occurs within a minute or two, but patients may remain pale, diaphoretic and mildly hypotensive for several more minutes. The likelihood of fainting is reduced by measures that lower stress in those awaiting vaccination, such as short waiting times, comfortable room temperature, preparation of vaccines out of view of recipients and privacy during the procedure. To reduce injuries during fainting spells those at risk are best vaccinated while seated.

Persons experiencing an anxiety spell may appear fearful, pale and diaphoretic and complain of lightheadedness, dizziness and numbness, as well as tingling of the face and extremities. Hyperventilation is usually evident. Treatment consists of reassurance and rebreathing using a paper bag until symptoms subside.

Breath-holding spells occur in some young children when they are upset and crying hard. The child is suddenly silent but obviously agitated. Facial flushing and peri-oral cyanosis deepen as breath-holding continues. Some spells end with resumption of crying but others end with a brief period of unconsciousness during which breathing resumes. Similar spells may have been evident in other circumstances. No treatment is required beyond reassurance of the child and parents.

In the case of anaphylaxis, changes develop over several minutes and usually involve multiple body systems (affecting the skin, respiration, circulation). Unconsciousness is rarely the sole manifestation of anaphylaxis. It occurs only as a late event in severe cases.

The cardinal features of anaphylaxis are

■ itchy, urticarial rash (in over 90% of cases);

■ progressive, painless swelling (angioedema) about the face and mouth, which may be preceded by itchiness, tearing, nasal congestion or facial flushing;

■ respiratory symptoms, including sneezing, coughing, wheezing, and laboured breathing; upper airway swelling (indicated by hoarseness and/or difficulty swallowing) possibly causing airway obstruction;

■ hypotension, which generally develops later in the illness and can progress to cause shock and collapse.

An inconstant early feature is swelling and urticarial rash at the injection site. This is more likely to be evident with vaccines injected subcutaneously than intramuscularly.

Anaphylaxis is described as mild or early when signs are limited to urticarial rash and injection site swelling. At this stage symptoms may arise from other systems (e.g., sneezing, nasal congestion, tearing, coughing, facial flushing) but are associated with minimal dysfunction. Features of severe disease include obstructive swelling of the upper airway, marked bronchospasm and hypotension.

Management of anaphylaxis

The following steps describe the management of anaphylaxis. Steps 1 to 5 are meant to be done rapidly or simultaneously. The priority is prompt administration of epinephrine (step 5), which should not be delayed if earlier steps cannot quickly be completed.

1. Call for assistance, including an ambulance.

2. Place the patient in a recumbent position (elevating the feet if possible).

3. Establish an oral airway if necessary.

4. Place a tourniquet (when possible) above the site of vaccination. Release for 1 minute every 3 minutes. This delays absorption of the vaccine until the medication takes effect. It can be stopped as symptoms subside.

5. Promptly administer 0.01 mL/kg (maximum 0.5 mL) of aqueous epinephrine 1:1,000 by subcutaneous or intramuscular injection in the opposite limb to that in which the vaccination was given. Speedy intervention is of paramount importance: failure to use epinephrine promptly is more dangerous than using it improperly.

The subcutaneous route of epinephrine injection is appropriate for mild or early cases, and a single injection is usually sufficient. Severe cases should receive intramuscular injections because they lead more quickly to generalized distribution of the drug.

Dosing can be repeated twice at 20-minute intervals if necessary, again avoiding the limb in which the vaccination was given. A different limb is preferred for each dose to maximize drug absorption. Severe reactions could require these repeat doses to be given at shorter intervals (10 to 15 minutes).

The epinephrine dose should be carefully determined. Calculations based on body weight are preferred when weight is known. Recording the weight of children before routine immunization is recommended when feasible. Excessive doses of epinephrine can add to patients' distress by causing palpitations, tachycardia, flushing and headache. Although unpleasant, such side effects pose little danger. Cardiac dysrhythmias may occur in older adults but are rare in otherwise healthy children.

When body weight is not known the dose of aqueous epinephrine 1:1,000 can be approximated from the subject's age (Table 3).

The anaphylactic state in patients receiving beta-adrenergic antagonist therapy (for elevated blood pressure) will be more resistant to epinephrine therapy.

Since anaphylaxis is rare, epinephrine vials and other emergency supplies should be checked on a regular basis and replaced if outdated.

Table 3
Appropriate Dose of Epinephrine According to Age

Age	Dose	
2 to 6 months*	0.07 mL	(0.07 mg)
12 months*	0.10 mL	(0.10 mg)
18 months* to 4 years	0.15 mL	(0.15 mg)
5 years	0.20 mL	(0.20 mg)
6-9 years	0.30 mL	(0.30 mg)
10-13 years	0.40 mL†	(0.40 mg)
≥ 14 years	0.50 mL†	(0.50 mg)

* Doses for children between the ages shown should be approximated, the volume being intermediate between the values shown or increased to the next larger dose, depending on practicability.
† For a mild reaction a dose of 0.3 mL can be considered.

6. If the vaccine was injected subcutaneously, an additional dose of 0.005 mL/kg (maximum 0.3 mL) of aqueous epinephrine 1:1,000 can be injected into the vaccination site to slow absorption. This should be given shortly after the initial dose of epinephrine (Table 3) in moderate to severe cases. It is generally not repeated. Local injection of epinephrine into an intramuscular vaccination site is contraindicated because it dilates vessels and speeds absorption.

7. As an adjunct to epinephrine, a dose of diphenhydramine hydrochloride (Benadryl®) can be given. It should be reserved for patients not responding well to epinephrine or to maintain symptom control in those who have responded (epinephrine being a short-acting agent), especially if transfer to an acute care facility cannot be effected within 30 minutes. Oral treatment is preferred for conscious patients who are not seriously ill because Benadryl® is painful when given intramuscularly. This drug has a high safety margin, making precise dosing less important. The approximate doses of diphenhydramine HCl (Benadryl® for injection 50 mg/mL solution) are shown in Table 4.

8. Monitor vital signs and reassess the situation frequently, to guide medication use.

9. Arrange for rapid transport to an emergency department.

   For all but the mildest cases of anaphylaxis, patients should be hospitalized overnight or monitored for at least 12 hours.

Table 4
Appropriate Dose of Diphenhydramine Hydrochloride (50 mg/mL Solution)

Age	Dose	
< 2 years	0.25 mL	(12.5 mg)
2-4 years	0.50 mL	(25.0 mg)
5-11 years	1.00 mL	(50.0 mg)
≥ 12 years	1.00-2.00 mL	(50-100 mg)

SELECTED REFERENCE

Thibodeau JL. *Office management of childhood vaccine-related anaphylaxis*. Can Fam Phys 1993;40:1602-10.

Live Vaccines

Immunizing agents that contain living microorganisms (measles, rubella, mumps, BCG, yellow fever and oral polio vaccines) should not generally be given to patients with conditions in which immune mechanisms are impaired, including the following:

1. patients with immune deficiency diseases such as hypogammaglobulinemia or combined immunodeficiency;

2. patients with altered immune status due to diseases such as leukemia, lymphoma or other generalized malignant disease;

3. patients with immunosuppression induced by therapy with corticosteroids, antimetabolites, alkylating drugs or radiation.

For immunization of immunocompromised persons see page 14.

Immunization and Pregnancy

Immunization of a pregnant woman may be indicated when the risk of the disease outweighs the risk of the vaccine both for the mother and the fetus. When this condition is not met, any vaccination should be deferred until after delivery. There is no evidence to suggest that pregnant women are at greater risk of allergic reactions than other people, but the occurrence of a severe anaphylactic reaction and its treatment can have dramatic adverse consequences for the fetus. Fever is a possible reaction to many vaccines, and epidemiologic and animal studies indicate that maternal hyperthermia during the first trimester of pregnancy may be teratogenic. The magnitude of this risk is not known precisely. For live vaccines, there is a risk of fetal infection, but specific fetal damage has not been reported from administration of the currently used vaccines during pregnancy. Inactivated vaccines and toxoids are usually considered safe for the fetus. There is no known risk to the fetus from passive immunization of pregnant women with immune globulin preparations.

SELECTED REFERENCES

Lynberg MC, Khourg MJ, Lu X et al. *Maternal flu, fever, and the risk of neural defects: a population-based case-control study.* Am J Epidemiol 1994;140:244-55.

Milunsky A et al. *Maternal heat exposure and neural tube defects.* JAMA 1992;268:882-85.

Smith MS et al. *The induction of neural tube defects by maternal hyperthermia: a comparison of the guinea-pig and human.* Neuropathol Appl Neurobiol 1992;18:71-80.

Tikkanen J, Heinonen OP. *Maternal hyperthermia during pregnancy and cardio-vascular malformations in the offspring.* Eur J Epidemiol 1991;7:628-35.

Immunization and Breast-feeding
Breast-feeding does not adversely affect immunization of the infant with either live or killed vaccines. Infants who are breast-fed should receive all recommended vaccinations at the usual times.

Lactating mothers who have not received the recommended immunizations may safely be given rubella and other routinely used vaccines postpartum.

Immunization of Children with Neurologic Disorders
Children with neurologic disorders can undergo routine vaccinations. For those with seizure disorders that might be exacerbated by fever, prophylactic doses of acetaminophen (15 mg/kg) can be used.

Vaccination in Immunocompromised Hosts
The number of immunocompromised individuals in Canadian society is steadily increasing for a wide variety of reasons (outlined in Table 5). The number of vaccines to which an immunocompromised individual is likely to be exposed is also increasing because of the enlarging spectrum of vaccines available, the inclusion of more vaccines in universal programs, the renewed efforts to fully immunize adolescents, adults and the elderly and the ease with which individuals with significant illness can now travel.

Table 5
Factors that Contribute to an Increased Number of Immunocompromised Individuals in the Canadian Population

More sophisticated understanding of "normal" and altered immunity • IgG subclass deficiencies • mannose-binding protein deficiency • cytokine receptor deficiencies
Recognition of subtle immunodeficiencies associated with • chronic illnesses (e.g., diabetes, cirrhosis) • extremes of age
The HIV pandemic
Expanding range of illnesses treated with immunomodulatory agents • autoimmune diseases • inflammatory conditions
Accumulation of long-term survivors after organ transplantation and cancer
Increased use of ablative therapy for cancer and other conditions
Accumulation of individuals with absent or dysfunctional spleens

As a result of these factors, questions dealing with vaccination in immuno-compromised hosts are increasing rapidly in both frequency and complexity. Still further complexity is added by the fact that the degree to which individuals are immunocompromised may vary over time (e.g., in those with HIV or patients who have undergone bone marrow transplantation [BMT]) and the observation that many of these hosts respond poorly to "routine" vaccination. The decision to recommend for or against any particular vaccine will depend upon a careful, case-by-case analysis of the risks and benefits. Analysis of benefit is often limited by the paucity of data on the effectiveness of vaccination in these diverse conditions. There is potential for significant morbidity and mortality in both the under-vaccination and over-vaccination of immunocompromised hosts. Vaccination of individuals who are significantly immunocompromised should be performed or supervised by personnel with special training.

General principles
Several general principles apply to the vaccination of immunocompromised individuals.

■ Maximize benefit while minimizing harm

■ Make no assumptions about susceptibility or protection (a history of childhood infection or previous vaccination may be irrelevant)

Part 1 – General Considerations

15

- Vaccinate at the time when maximum immune response can be anticipated:
  - vaccinate early when immunologic decline is predictable
  - delay vaccination if the immunodeficiency is transient (if this can be done safely)
  - stop or reduce immunosuppression to permit better vaccine response
- Consider the vaccination environment broadly:
  - family of the vaccinee (e.g., spread of oral poliovirus from family members)
  - vaccination status of both donor and recipient in BMT
  - vaccination status of family and caregivers in case individual needs protection (e.g., against influenza)
- Avoid live vaccines unless:
  - data are available to support their use
  - the risk of natural infection is greater than the risk of vaccination
- Monitor subjects carefully and boost actively:
  - the degree and duration of vaccine-induced immunity are often reduced
  - some vaccine-strain organisms can persist for years in compromised hosts
- Consider the use of passive immunizing agents:
  - serum immune globulin (IG)
  - intravenous immune globulin (IGIV)
  - the several "pathogen-specific" IG that are available (e.g., varicella Ig, tetanus IG)

Approach to vaccination of immunodeficient hosts (Table 6)

The approach to vaccinating individuals with immunodeficiency varies with the precise nature of the defect. Additional considerations include the age of the individual (together with the types of vaccines and the relative urgency of vaccination) and factors that influence the risk of exposure to the different pathogens (e.g., endemic, epidemic, professional, travel). The most common situations are discussed next by broad category of immunodeficiency.

Otherwise "normal" subjects with chronic illness or advanced age

These individuals are not necessarily more susceptible to vaccine-preventable diseases but are more likely to suffer significant morbidity and mortality from these infections. There are no contra-indications to the use of any vaccine in these people. Particular attention should be paid to annual influenza vaccination, pneumococcal vaccination with a possible booster dose after 5 years and at least one Td booster in adulthood (the data supporting a need for Td boosting every 10 years are limited). Hepatitis A and/or B immunization may be appropriate in people with chronic liver disease since they are at risk of fulminant hepatitis. Accelerated vaccination schedules or early vaccination should be considered in individuals who are likely to undergo solid organ transplantation (e.g., hepatitis B vaccination in subjects with deteriorating renal function). Immune responses to vaccines will be suboptimal in many of these individuals. Evidence is accumulating that individuals with chronic disease may be induced to respond with higher doses of some vaccine antigens (e.g., hepatitis B in patients receiving dialysis).

Splenic disorders

Asplenia or hyposplenism may be congenital, surgical or functional. A number of conditions not typically thought of as immunocompromising can lead to functional hyposplenism. These include sickle cell anemia, thalassemia major, essential thrombocytopenia, celiac disease and inflammatory bowel disease. There are no contra-indications to the use of any vaccine in people with these conditions. Particular attention should be paid to ensuring optimal protection against ubiquitous encapsulated bacteria (*Streptococcus pneumoniae, Haemophilus influenzae*), to which these individuals are highly susceptible. They may also benefit from annual influenza vaccination. Meningococcal vaccination (quadrivalent) is essential in hyposplenic and asplenic individuals who reside in or travel to areas of endemicity. There are limited data addressing the issues of efficacy and timing of booster doses for plain polysaccharide vaccines. The 23-valent pneumococcal vaccine should be recommended for all people who received the original 14-valent product. This vaccine can be re-administered safely after 5 years. Although meningococcal vaccination can be boosted safely every 2-3 years, recent Canadian data suggest that the antibody response to some of the component polysaccharides may be very limited. In young patients (< 10 years of age), it may be prudent to verify the presence of antibodies directed against *H. influenzae* and revaccinate as needed. Careful attention should be paid to vaccination status when elective surgical splenectomy is planned so that all of the necessary vaccines can be delivered at least 2 weeks before removal of the spleen.

Congenital immunodeficiency states

This is a varied group of conditions including defects in antibody production (e.g., agammaglobulinemia, isotype and IgG subclass deficiencies, hyper-IgM syndromes), complement deficiencies, defects in one or more aspects of cell-mediated immunity (CMI) and mixed deficits. Individuals with defects in antibody and complement have unusual susceptibility to the encapsulated bacteria and enteroviruses (e.g., polio, coxsackie and echoviruses), and those with mixed and T cell defects are particularly susceptible to intracellular pathogens (virtually all viruses and some bacteria, fungi and parasites). Although the defects and susceptibility patterns are very different, the approach to vaccination is quite similar for these people. Component and inactivated vaccines can and should be administered in all of these conditions despite the fact that many of the individuals will respond poorly, if at all. Live vaccines are generally not recommended although limited clinical data suggest that MMR can be administered without undue risk in people with pure antibody defects.

Antibody defects: Particular attention should be given to ensuring that vaccination is carried out against pneumococcal disease, *Haemophilus influenzae* and possibly meningococcal disease in these individuals. Oral poliovirus vaccine must not be used in the affected individual or any of his/her family members. Other live vaccines may be considered on a case-by-case basis after a thorough review of the risks and benefits. As a general rule, these people can be protected from many of the vaccine-preventable infections by the use of IGIV or pathogen-specific IG preparations. Inactivated vaccines should be timed for administration during the nadirs of IGIV-supported immunoglobulin levels.

T cell, natural killer and mixed CMI-antibody defects: Live vaccines (including BCG) are contraindicated. Inadvertent live vaccine administration and exposures to natural infections must be dealt with by rapid administration of IG or pathogen-specific IG as well as appropriate anti-viral/anti-bacterial treatment if available.

Granulocyte defects: There are no contraindications to the use of any of the currently available vaccines.

Long-term steroids/azothiaprine/cyclosporine/cyclophosphamide

Long-term immunosuppressive therapy is used for organ transplantation and an increasing range of chronic infectious and inflammatory conditions (e.g., inflammatory bowel disease, collagen vascular disease). These therapies alone or in combination have their greatest impact on cell-mediated immunity, although help for T cell-dependent antibody production can also be reduced. Ideally, all appropriate vaccines/boosters should be administered to individuals undergoing such therapy at least 10-14 days before the initiation of therapy. If this cannot be done safely, vaccination should be delayed until at least 3 months after immunosuppressive drugs have been stopped or until such therapy is at the lowest possible level. There is no contraindication to the use of any inactivated vaccine in these people, and particular attention should be paid to the completion of childhood immunizations, annual influenza vaccination and pneumococcal vaccination (with a boost at 5 years). Active verification of immune status and aggressive reimmunization may be important for some subjects (e.g., against *Haemophilus influenzae* in children < 10 years of age, hepatitis B for renal transplant recipients). Live vaccines are generally contraindicated in this setting, although it is likely that individuals taking low maintenance doses of immunosuppressive drugs could receive them safely if the risk of natural infection is significant (e.g., yellow fever vaccination for travel to an area with an epidemic). On the theoretic grounds that vaccine-induced immunostimulation might trigger an anti-transplant response, some centres choose to avoid vaccines and rely on immunoglobulin preparations with or without appropriate antimicrobial drugs.

Steroids: Only high dose, systemic steroids interfere with vaccine-induced immune responses (e.g., $\geq$ 2mg/kg of prednisone/day for more than 2 weeks or $\geq$ 60 mg prednisone/day in an adult). Topical and inhaled steroids have no known impact on oral or injected vaccines. A period of at least 3 months should elapse between high dose steroid use and administration of both inactivated and component vaccines (to ensure immunogenicity) and live vaccines (to reduce the risk of dissemination).

Immunoablative therapy (e.g., cancer chemotherapy, total body irradiation, bone marrow transplantation)

If time permits, careful consideration must be given to pre-ablation vaccination status in the patient and, in the case of allogeneic BMT, the donor. It is well established that disease and vaccination histories in both the host and the donor (i.e., adoptive transfer) can influence post-ablation/transplantation immunity. Although the argument for systematic vaccination of these subjects is compelling, there are relatively few data on important vaccination-related questions after ablative therapies (e.g., optimal timing, requirement for boosters, overall efficacy, cost-benefit). A recent U.S. national survey of transplantation services has demonstrated striking inconsistencies in the application of pre- and post-ablative vaccination policies.

General principles in this setting are as follows:

- Live vaccines are contraindicated before ablation when significant marrow infiltration is present.

- All appropriate vaccines and boosters should be administered at least 10-14 days before ablative therapy if this can be accomplished without delaying the initiation of chemotherapy.

- In allogeneic BMT, consider administration of all appropriate vaccines and boosters to the donor at least 10-14 days before the marrow harvest (e.g.,Td).

- Wait at least **24 months** after ablative therapy before administering live vaccines and then only if there is no ongoing immune suppressive treatment or graft-versus-host disease (GVHD) **(note: BCG is contraindicated at all times)**.

- Inactivated or component vaccines can usually be given within 12 months after transplantation although responses to many vaccines are suboptimal. The primary immunization schedule should be re-initiated at 12 months after transplantation in children whose original schedule was disrupted. Revaccination should also be offered to older children and adults using either a full primary series or at least two booster doses.

- Consider documentation of responses to the most important pathogens (e.g., measles, varicella).

Table 6
Vaccination of Individuals with Immunodeficiency

Vaccine	HIV/AIDS	Severe immuno-deficiency	Solid organ transplantation	BMT	Chronic disease age/alcoholism	Hypo- or asplenia
Inactivated/Component Vaccines						
DPT (Td)	Routine use*	Routine use	Recommended†	Recommended	Routine use	Routine use
IPV	Routine use	Routine use	Recommended	Recommended	Routine use	Routine use
Hib	Routine use	Routine use	Recommended	Recommended	Routine use	Recommended (confirm response in children <10)
Influenza	Recommended	Recommended	Recommended	Recommended	Recommended	Recommended
Pneumococcal	Recommended	Recommended	Recommended	Recommended	Recommended	Recommended
Meningococcal	Use if indicated	Use if indicated	Use if indicated	Use if indicated	Use if indicated	Use if indicated
Hepatitis A	Recommended (gay men, IVDU)	Use if indicated	Use if indicated	Use if indicated	Recommended (chronic liver disease)	Use if indicated
Hepatitis B	Recommended (gay men, IVDU)	Routine use	Routine use	Routine use	Recommended (chronic liver or renal disease)	Routine use

Vaccine	HIV/AIDS	Severe immuno-deficiency	Solid organ transplantation	BMT	Chronic disease age/alcoholism	Hypo- or asplenia
Live Vaccines						
MMR	Routine use ‡ (if no significant compromise)	Contraindicated	Consider at 24 mo (min. suppressive Rx)	Consider at 24 mo (no suppressive Rx, no GVHD)	Use if indicated	Use if indicated
OPV	Contraindicated (use IPV instead)	Contraindicated (use IPV instead)	Contraindicated (use IPV instead)	Contraindicated (use IPV instead)	If indicated use IPV	If indicated use IPV
Varicella	Use if indicated (asymptomatic disease)	Contraindicated	Consider at 24 mo (min. suppressive Rx)	Consider at 24 mo (no suppressive Rx, no GVHD)	Use if indicated	Use if indicated
Oral typhoid	Contraindicated (use IM vaccine instead)	Contraindicated (use IM vaccine instead)	Contraindicated (use IM vaccine instead)	Contraindicated (use IM vaccine instead)	If indicated use IM	If indicated use IM
BCG	Contraindicated	Contraindicated	Contraindicated	Contraindicated	Use if indicated	Use if indicated
Yellow fever	Contraindicated	Contraindicated	Consider at 24 mo (no suppressive Rx, no GVHD)	Consider at 24 mo (no suppressive Rx, no GVHD)	Use if indicated	Use if indicated
Oral cholera	Contraindicated	Contraindicated	Contraindicated	Contraindicated	Use if indicated	Use if indicated

* Routine vaccination schedules should be followed with age-appropriate booster doses.

† Vaccination and/or revaccination recommended with or without verification of serologic response.

‡ Most HIV positive children can receive the first MMR vaccine without significant risk. Administration of the second MMR dose (particularly in adults) must be evaluated on a case-by-case basis.

Illnesses that progressively weaken the immune system (e.g., HIV, myelodysplasias)
There are no contraindications to the use of any vaccine (including BCG and MMR) early in the course of these illnesses if the patient is not significantly immunocompromised. However, the immune status of these individuals must be carefully assessed before vaccination. With progression of illness, the use of live vaccines becomes increasingly dangerous, and the risks and benefits of a particular vaccine (and the alternative therapies available) need to be carefully considered. Early vaccination is more effective in these conditions. There are no contraindications to the use of inactivated or component vaccines at any time. Particular attention should be paid to the completion of childhood immunizations, pneumococcal vaccination (with a booster dose at 5 years), annual influenza vaccination and serologic confirmation of response to *H. influenzae* type b vaccination in children < 10 years of age (with revaccination if necessary). Exposures to wild-type infections must be addressed promptly with pooled or specific Ig preparations with or without antimicrobial therapy, since the mortality rates among these patients can be very high (e.g., 50%-100% mortality from measles in AIDS patients). Concerns have been raised about transient increases in HIV viral load that can occur after a number of routine vaccinations. Although changes in viral load after wild-type, vaccine-preventable infections have not been studied, it is likely that the greater immune activation induced by the natural infections gives rise to similar or greater increases in viral load. Therefore, fears of transient increases in viral load should not prevent the administration of any appropriate vaccine. The only exception to this general rule would be an HIV-positive woman who has decided to breast-feed. In this case, the administration of appropriate vaccines to the mother should be delayed until after breastfeeding has stopped if this can be done without undue risk to the mother.

Immunocompromised travellers
Although the degree and range of risks can increase dramatically when an immunocompromised individual gets onto an airplane or boat, the basic principles outlined still apply. When a certificate of yellow fever vaccination is required but this vaccine is contraindicated, a letter of deferral should be supplied to the patient. Pretravel care for these individuals requires consultation between international health experts and specialists trained in the care of immunocompromised hosts.

SELECTED REFERENCES

ACP Task Force on Adult Immunization. *Immunizations for immunocompromised adults. Guide for adult immunization.* Third Edition. American College of Physicians, 1994;49-59.

Ambrosino DM, Molrine DC. *Critical appraisal of immunization strategies for prevention of infection in the compromised host.* Hematol Oncol Clin North Am 1993;7:1027-50.

Centers for Disease Control and Prevention. *Recommendations of the Advisory Committee on Immunization Practices (ACIP): use of vaccines and immune globulins in persons with altered immunocompetence.* MMWR 1993;42:1-18.

Chan CY, Molrine DC, Antin JH et al. *Antibody response to tetanus toxoid and* **Haemophilus influenzae** *type B conjugate vaccines following autologous peripheral blood stem cell transplantation (PBX).* Bone Marrow Transplant 1997;20:33-8.

Glesby MJ, Hoover DR, Farzadegan H, Margolick JB, Saah AJ. *The effect of influenza vaccination on human immunodeficiency virus type 1 load: A randomized, double-blind, placebo controlled study.* J Infect Dis 1996;174:1332-36.

Henning KJ, White MH, Sepkowitz KA, Armstrong D. *A national survey of immunization practices following allogenic bone marrow transplantation.* JAMA 1997;277:1148-51.

Hughes I, Jenney ME, Newton RW et al. *Measles encephalitis during immuno-suppressive treatment for acute lymphoblastic leukemia.* Arch Dis Child 1993;68:775-78.

Ljungman P. *Immunization in the immunocompromised host.* Curr Opin Infect Dis 1995;8:254-57.

Lout L. *Vaccination of the immunocompromised patient.* Biologicals 1997;25:231-6.

Parkkali T, Olander RM, Ruutu T et al. *A randomized comparison between early and late vaccination with tetanus toxoid vaccine after allegenic BMT.* Bone Marrow Transplant 1997;19:933-38.

Ridgeway D, Wolff LJ. *Active immunization of children with leukemia and other malignancies.* Leuk Lymphoma 1993;9:177-92.

Rosen HR, Sticrer M, Wolf HM, Eibl MM. *Impaired primary antibody responses after vaccination against hepatitis B in patients with breast cancer.* Breast Cancer Res Treatment 1992;23:233-40.

Shenep JL, Feldman S, Gigliotti F et al. *Response of immunocompromised children with solid tumors to a conjugate vaccine for* **Haemophilus influenzae** *type b.* J Pediatrics 1994;125:581-84.

Somani J, Larsn RA. *Reimmunization after allogenic bone marrow transplantation.* Am J Med 1995;98:389-98.

Working Party of the British Committee for Standards in Haematology — Clinical Haematology Task Force. *Guidelines for the prevention and treatment of infection in patients with an absent or dysfunctional spleen.* BMJ 1996;312:430-34.

Part 1 – General Considerations

23

Immunization of Persons with Hemophilia and Other Bleeding Disorders

Immunizations should be carried out using a fine gauge needle of appropriate length, followed by application of firm pressure, without rubbing, to the injection site for at least 5 minutes after the injection. Administration can be subcutaneous or intra-muscular depending on the product. If there is concern that an injection may stimulate bleeding, it can be scheduled shortly after administration of anti-hemophilia therapy.

Any patient with a bleeding disorder who needs plasma-derived products is at higher risk of contracting hepatitis A or B and should be offered the vaccine. Please refer to the appropriate chapter in the Guide for information on dosage.

Immunization of Infants Born Prematurely

Premature infants whose clinical condition is satisfactory should be immunized with full doses of vaccine at the same chronological age and according to the same schedule as full-term infants, regardless of birth weight. Antibody response to immunization is a function of post-natal age and not of maturity. In infants born prematurely, maternal antibody is present at lower titres and for a shorter duration than in mature infants.

The response to hepatitis B vaccine may be diminished in infants with birth weights below 2000 grams. Routine immunization of infants of mothers negative for hepatitis B surface antigen (HBsAg) should be delayed until the infant reaches 2000 grams or 2 months of age. Infants born to women who are HBsAg positive should receive hepatitis B immune globulin (HBIG) within 12 hours of birth and the appropriate dose of vaccine (see chapter on Hepatitis B Vaccine).

If the mother's status is unknown, the vaccine should be given in accordance with recommendations for the infant of an HBsAg positive mother. The maternal status should be determined within 12 hours and if the mother is HBsAg positive the infant should receive HBIG.

Preterm infants with chronic respiratory disease should be vaccinated against influenza annually in the fall when they reach 6 months of age. Delay of proper immunization has resulted in unnecessary deaths.

Timing of Vaccine Administration

For most products that require more than one dose or booster doses for full immunization, intervals between doses that are longer than those recommended do not lead to a reduction in final antibody concentrations. Therefore, *interruption of a recommended series of vaccinations for any reason does not necessitate starting the series over again, regardless of the interval elapsed.* However, there are exceptions, such as immunization against rabies. By contrast, doses given at less than the recommended interval may result in less than optimal antibody response and should not be counted as part of a primary series.

There are obvious practical advantages to giving more than one vaccine at the same time, especially in preparation for foreign travel or when there is doubt that the patient will return for further doses of vaccine. Most of the commonly used antigens can safely be given simultaneously. No increase in the frequency or severity of clinically significant side effects has been observed. The immune response to each antigen is generally adequate and comparable to that found in patients receiving these vaccines at separate times. Commercially prepared combinations of vaccines are convenient to use.

Unless specified by the manufacturer, inactivated vaccines should never be mixed in the same syringe. They can be given simultaneously, but at separate anatomic sites, consideration being given to the precautions that apply to each individual vaccine. No inactivated vaccine has been shown to interfere with the immune response to another inactivated vaccine; thus, no particular interval between inactivated vaccines need be respected.

Live parenteral vaccines should never be mixed in the same syringe, but may be administered simultaneously at different sites. One live parenteral vaccine may interfere with the effectiveness of another, and to minimize this possibility two or more live vaccines should preferably be administered either on the same day or be separated by an interval of at least 1 month. In travellers, the administration of oral typhoid and oral cholera vaccine should be separated by at least 8 hours.

Recent Administration of Human Immune Globulin Products

Passive immunization with products of human origin can interfere with the immune response to live viral vaccines. For measles vaccine, the recommended interval between immune globulin (IG) administration and subsequent vaccination varies from 3 to 10 or more months depending on the specific product given, as shown in Table 7.

For an optimum response to rubella or mumps vaccine given as individual components, there should be an interval of at least 3 months between administration of IG or blood products and vaccination. If given as combined MMR, then the longer intervals as recommended in Table 7 should be followed to ensure an adequate response to the measles vaccine component. For women susceptible to rubella who are given Rh immune globulins in the peripartum period, consult the chapter on rubella vaccine for specific recommendations regarding the timing of rubella vaccination.

Table 7
Guidelines for Interval between Administration of Immune Globulin Preparations or Blood, and Vaccines Containing Live Measles Virus

Product	Indication	Dose	Interval (months)

Immune globulin (IG)	Hepatitis A
	  Contact prophylaxis
	  International travel
	Measles prophylaxis
	  Normal contact
	  Immunocompromised contact
		0.02 mL/kg
		0.06 mL/kg
		
		0.25 mL/kg
		0.5 mL/kg
			3
			3
			
			5
			6

Intravenous immune globulin (IGIV)	Treatment of antibody deficiency	160 mg/kg 320 mg/kg 640 mg/kg	7 8 9
	Treatment of idiopathic thrombocytopenic purpura or Kawasaki disease	≥ 1280 mg/kg	≥ 10
Hepatitis B immune globulin (HBIG)	Hepatitis B prophylaxis	0.06 mL/kg	3
Rabies immune globulin (RIG)	Rabies prophylaxis	20 IU/kg	4
Tetanus immune globulin (TIG)	Tetanus prophylaxis	250 units	3
Varicella immune globulin (VZIG)	Varicella prophylaxis	125 units/ 10 kg	5
Washed red blood cells		10 mL/kg IV	0
Reconstituted red blood cells		10 mL/kg IV	3
Whole blood (Hct 36%)		10 mL/kg IV	6
Packed red blood cells		10 mL/kg IV	6
Plasma/platelet products		10 mL/kg IV	7
Intravenous respiratory syncytial virus immune globulin		75 mg/kg	10

If administration of an IG preparation becomes necessary **after** MMR vaccine or its individual component vaccines have been given, interference can also occur. If the interval between administration of any of these vaccines and subsequent administration of an IG preparation is less than 14 days, vaccination should be repeated at the interval indicated in the table unless serologic testing is performed and indicates that antibodies were produced. If the IG product is given more than 14 days after the vaccine, vaccination does not have to be repeated.

Because there is little interaction between IG preparations and inactivated vaccines, the latter can be given concurrently or after an IG preparation has been used. The vaccine and IG preparation should be given at different sites. There are no data to indicate that IG administration interferes with the response to inactivated vaccines, toxoids or the live vaccines for yellow fever, typhoid, cholera and polio.

Storage and Handling of Immunizing Agents

Immunizing agents are biological materials that are subject to gradual loss of potency from deterioration and denaturation. Such loss can be accelerated under certain conditions of transport, storage and handling. It may result in failure to stimulate an adequate immunologic response and, thus, in lower levels of protection against disease. Conditions that lead to loss of potency vary among products. Recommendations from the manufacturer and the National Advisory Committee on Immunization generally specify that most products should be stored at temperatures from +2° to +8° C. Exceptions exist (e.g., yellow fever, varicella and oral polio vaccines), for which recommended storage conditions are given in the manufacturers' product leaflets.

The term "cold chain" as used in this statement refers to all equipment and procedures needed to ensure that vaccines are protected from inappropriate temperatures and light, from the time of transport from the manufacturer to the time of administration. The effects of exposure to adverse environmental conditions such as freezing, heat and light are cumulative. Although data are available indicating that certain products remain stable at temperatures below and above +2° to +8° C for specified periods of time, mechanisms for monitoring cumulative exposures are rare. Additionally, different products are often transported and stored in the same container. Therefore, it is recommended that all biologicals for immunization be maintained at +2° to +8° C at all times unless otherwise specified in the product leaflet (e.g., freezing below -15° C required for varicella vaccine). Management of products that have been exposed to adverse conditions should be guided by specific instructions about these conditions from the vaccine supplier.

Monitoring of the vaccine cold chain is required to ensure that biologicals are being stored and transported at recommended temperatures. Testing of product potency or seroconversion rates as indicators of cold chain integrity are rarely feasible. Readers should refer to the Canadian National Guidelines for Vaccine Storage and Transportation, published in the Canada Communicable Disease Report in 1995, volume 21, pages 93-97.

Effects of environmental conditions and preparation factors on particular vaccines

For details of recommended storage and handling of specific products, refer to the manufacturer's product leaflet. Information in the leaflet may be updated periodically. The following general principles apply:

Multi-dose vials: Multi-dose vials should be removed from the refrigerator only to draw up the dose required, and should be replaced immediately.

Lyophilized (freeze dried) vaccines: Freeze dried vaccines (e.g., MMR, rubella, BCG, Act-HIB™) should be reconstituted immediately before use with the diluent provided for that purpose. If unused, reconstituted vaccines should be discarded at the end of the work day. Yellow fever vaccine should be used within 1 hour of reconstitution.

Light exposure: Measles, mumps, rubella and BCG vaccines should be protected from light at all times by storage of the vials in the cartons provided. After reconstitution, if vaccines are not used immediately they **must** be kept at +2° to +8° C and protected from light.

Freezing: The liquid inactivated and adsorbed vaccines should not be used if frozen. These include DPT, DT, DPT-polio, DT-polio, Td, Td-polio, hepatitis A and B vaccines, HbOC (HibTITER™), influenza and pneumococcal vaccines. Prior to use, liquid vaccines should be inspected for visible signs of freezing and should not be used if any indication of freezing is apparent or if a temperature recording device indicates that the vaccine was exposed to temperatures below -2° C.

Un-reconstituted live virus vaccines such as MMR and rubella vaccines may be used after they have been frozen, but repeated freezing and thawing should be avoided. Live oral poliovirus vaccine (OPV) is distributed frozen to central suppliers at temperatures below -14° C. OPV should not be refrozen after it has been thawed; thawed vaccine should be refrigerated and used within the time limit specified. Once opened, OPV dispensers may be used for up to 3 days, provided they are refrigerated at all times.

A positive "shake test" is the finding that liquid vaccine that has been frozen and then thawed contains granular particles immediately upon shaking. One half-hour after shaking, the supernatant is almost clear because granular particles rapidly settle on the bottom of the vial. The shake test may be positive after freezing of adsorbed vaccines (e.g., DPT polio, DPT, DT, Td and Td polio); however, a positive result does not consistently occur after freezing. Therefore, when other signs indicate that the vaccine may have been frozen, the vaccine should not be used, even if the shake test is negative.

Expiry: Vaccines should not be used beyond their expiry date. Those with dates specified as month/year are deemed to expire on the last day of the specified month.

All vaccines that cannot be used because of expiry or adverse environmental exposure should be returned to the source for appropriate recording of returns and disposal. Alternatively, they can be appropriately disposed of locally, and the quantities disposed of reported to the officials in charge of vaccine management in the jurisdiction. The vaccine supplier will be able to provide specific instructions.

Recommendations for personnel, equipment and procedures

The following recommendations are for all sites that dispense, store and handle immunizing agents (physicians' offices, health department clinics, pharmacies).

Personnel

1. Designate specific members of the staff to manage inventory and storage.

2. Train all office staff in appropriate storage and handling techniques.

3. Post instructions about vaccine storage and handling on or near the vaccine storage refrigerator.

Equipment

1. When transporting vaccines, use only insulated containers that have been shown to maintain temperature between +2° and +8° C. When ice packs are used, vaccine should not come into direct contact with the pack surface unless it is visibly sweating; crumpled paper can be used to prevent contact.

2. Use equipment according to the manufacturer's or supplier's instructions.

3. Purchase a full-size (domestic) non-frost-free refrigerator with a freezer compartment. A freezer compartment filled with ice cubes and freezer packs will help maintain the refrigerator compartment below 8° C in the event of a power failure. Half-size, under-the-counter "bar" models are more prone to temperature fluctuations during heavy use. Temperatures inside frost-free models may cycle widely.

4. Consult your local public health department about availability of monitoring devices and equipment for transport of vaccines.

5. Monitor refrigerator temperatures using a maximum-minimum thermometer.

6. Defrost the refrigerator regularly.

7. Obtain prompt servicing of the refrigerator if, after adjustment, the temperature remains or deviates below or above +2° to +8° C. If the refrigerator cannot be serviced, replace it.

Procedures

1. Inspect vaccines and accompanying temperature monitoring devices upon receipt for evidence of damage, freezing or excessive heat.

2. Store vaccines in a refrigerator immediately upon their arrival.

3. Place vaccines of the same type together. Place packages with earlier expiry dates at the front to promote use prior to expiry. Check stock monthly and remove expired vaccine.

4. Do not store vaccines on refrigerator doorshelves; use only the central part of the refrigerator.

5. Check the internal refrigerator thermometer twice daily and record temperatures.

6. Avoid frequent opening of the refrigerator, and avoid storing materials such as staff lunches in the same refrigerator as the vaccines.

7. Put plastic bottles of water or saline solution on doorshelves and/or the lower compartment of the refrigerator to stabilize internal temperatures and delay temperature rises in the event of a power or refrigerator failure.

8. Ensure that the wall outlet for the refrigerator is clearly marked "do not unplug" or is otherwise secured, to prevent accidental disconnection from power.

9. If your refrigerator malfunctions, transfer vaccines to a functioning refrigerator.

10. Promptly report vaccine exposures to temperatures below or above +2° to +8° C to your local public health department or vaccine manufacturer for advice on further handling of the exposed products.

Additional recommendations are for manufacturers and public health authorities responsible for shipping large quantities of immunizing agents:

Personnel

1. Ensure that vaccine packaging and transport staff receive appropriate training.

2. Be informed and available to provide advice about the management of vaccine exposed to temperatures below or above +2° to +8° C.

Equipment

1. Package vaccines for transport with clearly marked labels (e.g., "Vaccines – Refrigerate Immediately – Do Not Freeze") to prevent mishandling during transport and to facilitate prompt storage upon arrival.

2. Obtain information from the supplier about the ability of specific cold chain equipment to maintain temperatures between +2° and +8° C for a specified time period before the equipment is used. If data are unavailable, test the equipment using colorimetric monitors or continuous temperature monitoring devices. Without testing, a particular combination of packaging, insulated container and ice packs for transport of smaller quantities of vaccines cannot be reliably recommended. If using untested equipment, monitor the internal temperature of the container throughout transport.

3. For long distance transport during very cold ambient winter temperatures, use "ice packs" that have been chilled to +5° C for packing of vaccines that must not freeze.

Procedures

1. Monitor the transport of all large shipments of vaccines to and from the central provincial/territorial storage site using cold chain monitors or constant temperature recording devices. A variety of these devices are available. The choice of device will depend on the temperature range of interest, size of the shipment, duration of transport, logistics of required retrieval of a monitoring device, and its cost.

2. Monitor all transport over long distances (e.g., northern Canada) or over long periods, or when carriers are used that are not specifically designed for this purpose (e.g., airlines).

3. Periodically, evaluate the integrity of the cold chain of a sample of transport routes and storage sites. Correct problems when these are identified.

Research priorities

In Canada, few studies of the vaccine cold chain have been done. The adequacy of transport from central to regional and regional to local sites should be examined, with particular emphasis on long distances. Both summer and winter conditions should be considered, as should other causes of heating and freezing; the latter may be related to excessively cold weather, refrigerator temperatures or use of ice packs. Although problems can occur in central storage sites, priority should be given to studying local vaccine storage and handling.

Several studies have highlighted shortcomings in vaccine storage in physicians' offices. Vaccine storage is of greatest importance in Canadian jurisdictions that have physician-administered immunization programs. Different methods of enhancing health care worker practices related to vaccine handling should be evaluated in order to identify effective continuing medical education strategies and methods of increasing accountability for vaccine handling. Common practices include sending regular reminders to providers about vaccine storage and handling, and ensuring that recently licensed physicians new to the immunization program receive an information package. Adding vaccine storage and handling practices to those reviewed in quality of care assessments conducted by professional organizations should also be considered.

Manufacturers should undertake to conduct research on the stability of products below and above +2° to +8° C. Methods of monitoring, such as the use of colorimetric dots on vials of vaccines, should be explored. Economic analyses of technology to reduce vaccine wastage are also of interest.

SELECTED REFERENCES

Bishai DM, Bhatt S, Miller LT, Hayden GF. *Vaccine storage practices in pediatric offices.* Pediatrics 1992;89:193-96.

Brazeau M, Delisle G. *Cold chain study: danger of freezing vaccines.* CCDR 1993;19:33-8.

Casto DT, Brunell PA. *Safe handling of vaccines.* Pediatrics 1991;87:108-12.

Daniels S, Deshpande R, Naus M. *Evaluating the cold chain in Ontario: pilot study findings.* Public Health Epidemiol Rep Ont 1994;5:99-103.

Daniels S, Naus M. *Surveys of vaccine storage and handling in Ontario.* Public Health Epidemiol Rep Ont 1994;5:2-9.

Hardy M, Duclos P. *Vaccine storage and transportation in Canada: a pilot study on cold chain adherence.* Ottawa: Laboratory Centre for Disease Control, Health Canada, 1996.

Haworth EA, Booy R, Stirzaker L et al. *Is the cold chain for vaccines maintained in general practice?* BMJ 1993;307:242-44.

Jeremijenko A, Kelly H, Sibthorpe B, Attewell R. *Improving vaccine storage in general practice refrigerators.* BMJ 1996;312:1651-52.

Laboratory Centre for Disease Control, Health Canada. *National guidelines for vaccine storage and transportation.* CCDR 1995;21:93-7.

Stability of vaccines. WHO Bull 1990;68:118-20.

Thakker Y, Woods S. *Storage of vaccines in the community: Weak link in the cold chain?* BMJ 1992;304:756-58.

Woodyard E, Woodyard L, Alto WA. *Vaccine storage in the physician's office: a community study.* J Am Board Fam Pract 1995;8:91-4.

Immunization Technique

A. Injection site

The injection site should be carefully chosen to avoid major nerves and blood vessels. The best sites for subcutaneous or intramuscular vaccinations are the deltoid area or the anterolateral surface of the thigh. The latter is the site of choice for infants < 1 year of age because it provides the largest muscle. In children > 1 year of age, the deltoid is the preferred site since use of the anterolateral thigh results in frequent complaints of limping due to muscle pain. Children should be well restrained before injection.

The chosen site should be cleansed with a suitable antiseptic, such as isopropyl alcohol, which is allowed to dry on the skin before the injection is given. A separate, sterile needle and syringe should be used for each injection, and after use should be carefully disposed of in a container designed for this purpose.

Because of decreased immunogenicity reported with several vaccines, the buttock is not recommended as an immunization site, except when large volumes must be given, e.g., immunoglobulin. If the buttock is used, care must be exercised to avoid injury to the sciatic nerve by selecting a site in the upper, outer quadrant of the gluteus maximus and avoiding the central area.

B. Route of administration

Immunization should be given by the route of administration recommended by the manufacturer for each vaccine (see Table 8). An appropriate size and length of needle should be chosen to ensure that the vaccine is deposited within the proper tissue layer.

For subcutaneous injections, a 25 gauge, 1.6 cm (5/8 inch) needle is normally recommended. Insert it at a 45° angle into the tissues below the dermal layer of the skin.

For intramuscular injections, a longer needle is needed:

- at least 2.2 cm (7/8 inch) for those with little muscle mass, such as infants

- at least 2.5 cm (1 inch) for others

Needles of these lengths are recommended to avoid sterile abscess in subcutaneous tissue. There is no risk if the injection is too deep.

Pinch and raise the skin. After inserting the needle into the site, pull back on the plunger to determine whether the needle has entered a blood vessel. If so, withdraw the needle, select a new site, and use new materials.

For intradermal injections, choose a fine gauge needle (e.g., 26 or 27 gauge). With the bevel facing upwards, insert the needle under the outer layer of skin at an angle almost parallel to the skin. Insert the needle so that the bevel penetrates the skin. Inject the solution slowly for greater patient comfort and to avoid spraying and leaking. If done correctly, a bleb should appear in the skin at the injection site.

Table 8
Routes Of Administration

Vaccine	Preferred route of administration
BCG	Intradermal
Diphtheria toxoid (fluid)	Subcutaneous (SC)*
Diphtheria toxoid (adsorbed)†	Intramuscular (IM)
Hepatitis A	IM
Hepatitis B	IM
Haemophilus influenzae type b conjugate vaccine	IM
Influenza	IM; SC also permissible
Japanese encephalitis	SC
Meningococcal	SC
Measles	SC
MMR (measles, mumps, & rubella)	SC
MR (measles & rubella)	SC
Penta and Pentacel†	IM
Pertussis (monovalent acellular)	IM
Pertussis (monovalent whole cell)	SC
Plague	IM
Pneumococcal	IM, SC
Polio (IPV)	SC
Polio (OPV)	Oral
Rabies	IM
Rubella	SC
Tetanus toxoid (adsorbed)†	IM
Typhoid – oral	Oral
– Vi capsular	IM
Yellow fever	SC

* The vaccines that are listed as SC only should not be given intramuscularly because of the lack of efficacy data for this route.
† Any vaccine combination containing adsorbed antigen *must* be administered intramuscularly because of the risk of subcutaneous nodule or sterile abscess if it is administered subcutaneously. Examples are Td (tetanus & diphtheria), DaPT.

Immunization Records

Each person who is immunized should be given a permanent personal immunization record. Individuals should be instructed to retain the record, to produce it for updating whenever they receive a vaccination and, if possible, to keep it at hand (e.g., in the wallet). Parents should keep and maintain these records on behalf of their children. In the future, the immunizations received should be among the items of health information stored on the magnetic strip of the personal health card. Immunization registries for children should be developed, and appropriate data should be accessible to health providers through provincial/territorial health information systems; however, these do not replace the need for personal records.

Record-keeping procedures should facilitate the provision of immunization records. It is essential that the health care provider maintain a separate permanent record of the immunization history of each individual on the medical chart in a readily accessible section that is not to be thinned. Headings on this record should include

- the trade name of the product

- the date given

- dose

- site and route of administration

- manufacturer

- lot number

Manufacturers should be encouraged to produce tear-off labels for use on the chart when the product is administered, to assist with completeness of the record. The record should also include relevant serologic data (e.g., rubella serology) and documented episodes of adverse vaccine events.

Refer to the *National Guidelines for Childhood Immunization Practices* (page 48) for additional information about the use and maintenance of immunization records.

Immunization of Children with Inadequate Immunization Records

Many children present to physicians and public health officials with inadequate immunization records. In the absence of a standardized approach to the management of such children, they may be under- or over-immunized. The greatest concern with over-immunization relates to DPT-containing vaccines because of the potential for a higher incidence of local adverse reactions.

In every instance, an attempt should be made to obtain the child's immunization records from the previous health care provider. Written documentation of immunization is preferred; in some instances, telephoned information from the health care provider with the exact dates of vaccinations may be accepted. Parental oral reports of prior immunization correlate poorly with actual immunity and should not be accepted as evidence of immunization.

Although the potency of vaccines administered in other countries can be generally assumed to be adequate, immunization schedules vary and the age at immunization (e.g., against measles), number of doses and intervals between doses should be reviewed in determining the need for additional doses of vaccines. Mumps and rubella vaccines are in limited use in the developing world and in the countries of the former USSR, where measles vaccine alone is generally given. *Haemophilus influenzae* type b (Hib) conjugate vaccines are also in limited use.

Routine serologic testing of children without records to determine immunity is not practical. Instead, the following approach is recommended:

1. All children lacking written documentation of immunization should be started on a primary immunization schedule as appropriate for their age (see pages 46 and 47).

2. MMR, polio, Hib conjugate, hepatitis B and influenza vaccines can be given without concern about prior receipt of these vaccines because adverse effects of repeated vaccination have not been demonstrated.

3. Children in whom a serious adverse local reaction develops after administration of DPT, DTaP, DT or Td should be individually assessed before they receive additional doses of these vaccines. Serologic testing against diphtheria and tetanus may demonstrate immune status and may guide the need for continued immunization.

4. Pneumococcal vaccine should be given if indicated, as in most studies local reaction rates after revaccination were similar to rates after initial vaccination.

Consent Issues and Concerns Regarding Immunization

This section is a departure from the usual style of the Guide. While the chapters on vaccines and general recommendations are targeted to readers for scientific guidance, this chapter contains material to assist in counselling individuals and parents about some of the myths and misconceptions they may have heard regarding the safety and effectiveness of vaccinations. Rather than provide details and specific pieces of evidence, it is written in more general terms that have proved to be useful to patients or parents of patients.

Each vaccine chapter of this guide lists precautions, contraindications and adverse events that may be attributed to vaccine administration. Like any medical intervention, vaccination can never be completely without complications. These are evaluated prior to vaccine approval, and adverse effects are monitored on an ongoing basis once the vaccine is on the market. A very high benefit to risk ratio is demanded. The vast majority of vaccine reactions are benign and self-limited, and are due in part to a healthy (anticipated) response to the immunizing antigen. Serious adverse events are rare, and in many cases are coincidentally rather than causally associated with vaccine. Any adverse event related to a vaccine, however, takes on much greater importance relative to other drug products for a number of reasons:

- Vaccines are given to healthy individuals to prevent disease, and thus any side effects are manifest as overt illness in the absence of immediate benefit.

- The diseases that vaccines prevent are becoming less and less common, and many are less frequent than some of the side effects due to vaccination.

- Vaccines are administered to children on a routine basis, and in some provinces even mandated by legislation. Thus any harm may be felt to be "caused" by social pressure to be vaccinated.

Therefore, ongoing evaluation of the safety of vaccine products is critically important. This includes more than pre-market evaluation, and comprises both the monitoring and reporting of adverse events as well as the initiation of appropriate discussions with parents and vaccine recipients about any risks relative to benefits of immunization. The scope of such discussion differs in many ways from that which takes place before prescribing other drugs. This chapter provides some guidance and insight on counselling about the risks and benefits of immunization. It corrects a common misconception that vaccination is compulsory and outlines some of the more general concerns raised against vaccination. It also highlights the important distinction between causation and temporal association that is crucial in all discussions of vaccine safety. Finally, references are listed that may be helpful to both providers of vaccines and the individuals or the parents of children who receive them.

Consent and vaccinations

There is a duty in law to obtain informed consent for any medical procedure. Informed consent has been defined in the *Dictionary of Epidemiology* as "voluntary consent given by a subject or by a person responsible for a subject (e.g., a parent) for participation in an investigation, immunization program, treatment regimen, etc., after being informed of the purpose, methods, procedures, benefits, and risks. Awareness of risk is necessary for any subject to make an informed choice." This can be a challenge for providers of vaccines. In some countries, providers are required to distribute written information to vaccine recipients or their parents before immunization, but this is not the case in Canada.

The task of obtaining informed consent for vaccination is becoming more complex: appropriately, more and more questions are being asked about the vaccines being offered. Many questions relate to alleged dangers or lack of effectiveness of vaccines. These concerns are being circulated by those who oppose immunization, and though there are few of them their messages are often dramatic and misleading. Individuals and parents are increasingly exposed to them in print, on television and on the Internet. In public libraries and on magazine stands parents are confronted by many more publications about the dangers of vaccination than about their safety and effectiveness in controlling diseases that once disabled or killed in large numbers. It is important to acknowledge that vaccines have side effects and to discuss the reasons why vaccines are still important. The common misconceptions described later in this chapter form a basis from which to begin appropriate counselling about the importance of immunization relative to the rare incidence of serious side effects. These misconceptions also illustrate some of the ways misinformation about vaccines is propagated. They provide a framework for approaching other allegations raised against vaccination, and can assist in the informed consent process.

Compulsory immunizations

Some parents may feel that immunizations are compulsory or "forced". In reality, although certain provinces do have school entry vaccination requirements, these are not mandatory in the usual sense of the term. Rather, parents (or children, if old enough to give consent) are required to declare a choice of whether to have their child (or themselves) immunized or not. If they opt not to, their child may be excluded from school in the event of an outbreak. Therefore, the legislation is in place to ensure that all parents have an opportunity to bring their child's vaccination status up to date, preventing children from remaining unimmunized because of complacency or neglect. It ensures that school officials verify immunization status, and parents are given an opportunity to catch up if needed.

Adverse reactions and temporal coincidence

Infancy is a period of rapid growth and development. Serious illnesses and the initial presentation of pre-existing but undiagnosed conditions (such as developmental delay and neurologic disorders) are most common in the first year of life, a time when most vaccines are given. Thus symptoms close to a vaccination may be pure coincidence, or the vaccine may unmask the illness but is not actually responsible for causing it.

One of the most difficult concepts for people to appreciate is the distinction between causation and temporal association. An example is the alleged relationship between sudden infant death syndrome (SIDS) and vaccination. When an infant dies, the natural reaction is to blame an event that took place preceding the death. In reality, the incidence of SIDS in the absence of vaccination is still highest in the first 6 months of life. Since a baby receives three vaccinations during those first 6 months, by coincidence alone there is a strong chance that SIDS occurs after a vaccine is given. If SIDS were caused by vaccination, one would expect a higher proportion of cases to occur close in time to a vaccination than further removed. A number of well-controlled studies conducted during the 1980s found that the number of SIDS deaths temporally associated with DTP vaccination was within the range expected to occur by chance. Unfortunately, vaccination as a cause of SIDS continues to be a persistently disseminated misconception.

Misconceptions about vaccination: common issues and responses

The main difficulty immunization providers face in trying to respond to misconceptions is that the proponents of these myths are not only fully convinced of their position but have little difficulty advancing it zealously in the absence of any supporting data, or even with obvious data to the contrary. Vaccine advocates, on the other hand, tend to be less dogmatic, appreciating that these issues are complex. Therefore, when providers are faced with some difficult questions that do not have ready answers, people will tend to equate this uncertainty with lack of evidence to the contrary, and thus will lend more credence to the arguments against vaccination — not because they are correct, but because they are delivered with such blind conviction. The following four categories of misconceptions cover the more common myths challenging the safety and effectiveness of vaccines. There are considerably more that circulate extensively on the Internet and occasionally surface in the media; however, these four illustrate the range of concerns that people may present, and responding to them will open the door to encouraging people to develop a healthy scepticism of all messages regarding vaccine safety, whether extremely negative or unduly positive.

1. **Vaccines are useless, and in any case the diseases they purport to protect against have disappeared. Therefore, no one needs to be protected from them anyway.**

Part 1 – General Considerations

Many opponents to vaccination claim that vaccines do not really work since, as a result of better hygiene and sanitation, diseases had already begun to disappear before vaccines were introduced. In addition, since the diseases are absent or rare in Canada, protection is no longer required.

Improved socioeconomic conditions have undoubtedly had an impact on the incidence and outcome of disease. Better nutrition and the development of antibiotics and other treatments have increased survival rates among the sick; less crowded living conditions have reduced disease transmission; and lower birth rates have decreased the number of susceptible household contacts. However, sustained decreases only emerged and were temporally associated with the introduction of vaccines: it is hard to imagine that this would have occurred coincidentally in so many cases. A few examples illustrate this point:

1. Invasive disease due to *Haemophilus influenzae* type b, such as meningitis, was prevalent until just a few years ago. Sanitation is no better now than it was in 1990, so it is hard to attribute the virtual disappearance of Hib disease in children in recent years (from an estimated 2,000 cases a year prior to the availability of vaccine to less than 52 cases now) to anything but the introduction of routine immunization.

2. Varicella (chicken pox) has not diminished with the advent of modern sanitation, and almost all children get the disease some time in their childhood, just as they did 20 years ago, or 80 years ago.

3. Pertussis resurgence in several developed countries (Great Britain, Sweden and Japan) in which immunization levels for that disease were allowed to drop was dramatic and immediate. For example, in Japan a drop in vaccination rates from 70% to 20%-40% led to a jump in pertussis from 393 cases and no deaths in 1974 to 13,000 cases and 41 deaths in 1979. When immunization programs were restarted, the number of cases fell once again.

Another "proof" that vaccines do not work is allegedly demonstrated by the fact that the majority of people getting disease have been fully immunized. Although it is true that the majority of people getting vaccine-preventable diseases like measles have been fully immunized, this apparent paradox is explained as a direct result of the fact that very few people remain unimmunized in a population, and there are thus very few people susceptible because of lack of vaccination. Since no vaccine is 100% effective, over the years there is a buildup of vaccinated but susceptible individuals who outnumber those who are unvaccinated and susceptible. When an outbreak hits, it affects virtually all susceptible individuals. This means that essentially 100% of the unimmunized, who are by definition all susceptible, get disease. On the other hand, only a minority of the immunized will be infected, although the absolute number of vaccine failures usually outnumbers the number of unvaccinated susceptibles. It

40

sounds disconcerting to hear, for example, that "75% of those getting disease were fully vaccinated." This is true but very misleading: rather, the correct statement is to say that the disease affected "almost 100% of those who were not vaccinated, but less than 10% of those who were."

A final argument against immunization is that since vaccine-preventable diseases have been virtually eliminated from Canada, there is no need to be vaccinated. This belief can be dangerous for a number of reasons. When diseases are exclusively human or when immunization does not prevent carriage, introduction and spread can occur as long as the disease is present anywhere in the world. Also, by being protected, immunized individuals can protect those around them. There is a small number of people who cannot be vaccinated (because of severe allergies to vaccine components, for example) and a small number who do not respond to the vaccine. These people are susceptible to disease, and their only hope of protection is that people around them are immune and cannot pass disease along to them. Until diseases are eliminated entirely, vaccination must continue. Travellers can acquire these diseases when visiting other countries and unknowingly bring them into Canada. For diseases that are not exclusively human, such as tetanus, individuals will always be susceptible if not protected by vaccination.

2. **Vaccines cause many harmful side effects, including deaths, and they have long-term effects that we don't even know about. This proves that vaccines are not safe.**

Vaccines are actually very safe, despite statements to the contrary in much anti-vaccine literature, which often claim that vaccines are responsible for countless deaths and disability. The vast majority of adverse events associated with vaccines are minor and transient, like a sore arm or mild fever. These side effects can often be controlled by acetaminophen taken before or after vaccination, but sometimes cannot be completely avoided as they represent a normal response to the vaccine. More serious adverse events occur rarely, in the order of 1/1,000 to 1/1 million doses, and some are so rare that risk cannot be accurately assessed. This is the case for severe neurologic illness, including encephalopathy. Often, such illnesses attributed to a vaccine occur more frequently in individuals with no history of recent vaccination. As highlighted in the earlier section about temporal association, infancy is unfortunately a time when SIDS incidence is highest, in the order of 0.3 to 5 cases per 1,000. As well, neurologic illness or developmental problems first manifest themselves at that time, so vaccination may unmask or appear to be contributing to these events. With regard to vaccines causing death, there are so few deaths that could plausibly be attributed to vaccines that it is hard to assess the risk statistically. Each death reported to the Canadian Vaccine-Associated Adverse Events Surveillance System is evaluated to determine whether it is truly a vaccine-related problem; none of the deaths reported has occurred in normally healthy children without underlying disease. Similarly, in a comprehensive assessment of whether vaccines can lead to death, the Institute of

Medicine reviewers could not hypothesize a mechanism by which a vaccine could cause death other than by vaccine-strain viral infection or an adverse event that itself is causally related to vaccine administration. They found no reports of death in the literature or case reports submitted to the U.S. voluntary reporting system that could not be explained by at least one of these two mechanisms.

With regard to long-term effects, many vaccines have been in use for decades with no evidence of any long-term adverse effects. Allegations that vaccination causes autism, seizure disorders, cancer or Crohn's disease, among others, have never been substantiated. It is true that there is a paucity of formal studies on the long-term side effects of vaccination, but there is similarly no conclusive scientific proof of the allegations listed above. There will always be articles in the press or medical journals that report possible poor outcomes as a result of vaccination. Reports in medical journals are sometimes preliminary findings to stimulate further work and to exchange information. It is necessary to assess many sources before drawing final conclusions. Articles in some newspapers and magazines are often written from a very biased viewpoint. Their manner of presenting the data can be misleading and must be interpreted with caution.

In all the discussion of the safety of vaccines, however, looking at risk alone is not enough — one must always look at both risks and benefits. Even one serious adverse effect in a million doses of vaccine cannot be justified if there is no benefit from the vaccination. If there were no vaccines, however, there would be many more cases of disease, and along with them more serious side effects, including death. The examples from countries that have stopped or decreased their immunization programs have illustrated this fact time and again. To have a medical intervention as effective in preventing disease as vaccination and not to use it would be medically unethical.

3. **Giving a child multiple vaccinations for different diseases at the same time increases the risk of harmful side effects and can overload the immune system.**
   Some people feel that vaccine-preventable diseases are part of growing up, that vaccination is unnecessary and harmful to the normal process of development, and that vaccines are not "natural". However, there is no evidence to support the argument that such illnesses are necessary for the normal development of the immune system. Also, children are exposed to many foreign antigens every day: routine consumption of food introduces new bacteria into the body, and numerous bacteria live in the mouth and nose, exposing the immune system to still more antigens. An upper respiratory viral infection exposes a child to between 4 and 10 antigens, and a case of streptococcal throat infection to between 25 and 50. In the face of these normal events, it seems unlikely that the number of separate antigens contained in childhood vaccines represents an appreciable added burden on the immune system. There is no evidence that stimulating the immune system risks response fatigue, akin to overworking muscles. Indeed, available scientific data show no adverse effects on the normal

childhood immune system of simultaneous vaccinations with multiple vaccines. If it is possible to give several vaccinations at the same time it will mean fewer office visits for vaccinations, which saves parents both time and money and may be less traumatic for the child.

4. Alternatives to immunization can decrease the incidence of disease

Some of those who feel that vaccine-preventable diseases are an important part of growing up also believe that they can be prevented by adhering to optimal healthy lifestyles and using complementary medicine products to prevent or treat illness. There is no evidence that any of this works; instead, it is the reduced exposure to these illnesses (through vaccination of others) that gives a false impression of success. In outbreak situations, those not immunized consistently have much higher attack rates than those immunized, as illustrated in the example given earlier.

Conclusion

Providing a medical intervention that carries risk, however small, to healthy individuals brings with it a different set of challenges. In the case of immunization, although generations past have embraced this intervention as a miracle (and detractors, though present, had a minor voice), vaccines are now a victim of their own success and are being increasingly challenged from a number of fronts. Rapid and unchallenged communications spread misinformation as fast as or faster than accurate information, making the truth more difficult to distinguish.

Through providing vaccines in a climate of appropriate informed consent, and careful and timely counselling, including correction of the common misconceptions that are circulating, immunization will maintain its status as one of the most effective preventive maneuvers in medicine.

SELECTED REFERENCES

Freed GL, Katz SL, Clark SJ. *Safety of vaccinations. Miss America, the media, and public health* [see comments]. JAMA 1996;276:1869-72.

Freeman TR, Bass MJ. *Determinants of maternal tolerance of vaccine-related risks.* Family Pract 1992;9:36-41.

Howson CP, Howe CJ, Fineberg HV, eds. *Adverse effects of pertussis and rubella vaccines.* Institute of Medicine. Washington DC: National Academy Press, 1991.

Last J. *A dictionary of epidemiology.* 2nd edition. New York: Oxford University Press, 1988.

Stratton KR, Howe CJ, Johnston RB, eds. *Adverse events associated with childhood vaccines: evidence bearing on causality.* Institute of Medicine. Washington, DC: National Adademy Press, 1994.

Guide for Parents

Canadian Paediatric Society. *Your child's best shot: a parent's guide to vaccination.* Ottawa: Canadian Paediatric Society, 1997.

Part 2
RECOMMENDED IMMUNIZATION FOR INFANTS, CHILDREN AND ADULTS

A.   Recommended Immunization Schedules for Infants and Children

Few measures in preventive medicine are of such proven value and as easy to implement as routine immunization against infectious diseases. Immunization carried out as recommended in the following schedules will provide good basic protection for most children against the diseases shown.

Both live and inactivated polio vaccines have been used in Canada with equal success in preventing the occurrence of paralytic poliomyelitis, but inactivated vaccine is now preferred.

Following a standard schedule ensures complete and adequate protection. However, modifications of the recommended schedule may be necessary because of missed appointments or intercurrent illness. Interruption of a recommended series does not require starting the series over again, regardless of the interval elapsed.

Similar vaccines are now available from different manufacturers, but they may not be identical. It is therefore essential for the user to read the appropriate chapter in this Guide as well as the manufacturer's package insert.

Table 1
Routine Immunization Schedule for Infants and Children

Age at vaccination	DTaP[1]	Inactivated polio vaccine	Hib[2]	MMR	Td[3]	Hep B[4] (3 doses)
Birth						
2 months	X	X	X			Infancy
4 months	X	X	X			
6 months	X	(X)[5]	X			
12 months				X		or
18 months	X	X	X	(X)[6] or		
4-6 years	X	X		(X)[6]		
14-16 years					X	preadolescence (9-13 yrs)

DTaP	Diphtheria, tetanus, pertussis (acellular) vaccine
Hib	*Haemophilus influenzae* type b conjugate vaccine
MMR	Measles, mumps and rubella vaccine
Td	Tetanus and diphtheria toxoid, "adult type"
Hep B	Hepatitis B vaccine

Table 2
Routine Immunization Schedule for Children < 7 Years of Age
Not Immunized in Early Infancy

Timing	DtaP[1]	Inactivated polio vaccine	Hib	MMR	Td[3]	Hep B[4] (3 doses)
First visit	X	X	X	X[7]		
2 months later	X	X	(X)[8]	(X)[6]		
2 months later	X	(X)[5]				Preadolescence
6-12 months later	X	X	(X)[8]			
4-6 years[9]	X	X				(9-13 yrs)
14-16 years					X	

46

Table 3
Routine Immunization Schedule for Children ≥ 7 Years of Age
Not Immunized in Early Infancy

Timing	Td[3]	Inactivated polio vccine	MMR	Hep B[4] (3 doses)
First visit	X	X	X	
2 months later	X	X	(X)[6]	Preadolescence
6-12 months later	X	X		(9-13 yrs)
10 years later	X			

Notes:

1. DTaP (diphtheria, tetanus, acellular or component pertussis) vaccine is the preferred vaccine for all doses in the vaccination series, including completion of the series in children who have received ≥ 1 dose of DPT (whole cell) vaccine.
2. Hib schedule shown is for PRP-T or HbOC vaccine. If PRP-OMP, give at 2, 4 and 12 months of age.
3. Td (tetanus and diphtheria toxoid), a combined adsorbed "adult type" preparation for use in persons ≥ 7 years of age, contains less diphtheria toxoid than preparations given to younger children and is less likely to cause reactions in older persons.
4. Hepatitis B vaccine can be routinely given to infants or pre-adolescents, depending on the provincial/territorial policy; three doses at 0, 1 and 6 month intervals are preferred. The second dose should be administered at least 1 month after the first dose, and the third dose should be administered at least 4 months after the first dose, and at least 2 months after the second dose.
5. This dose is not needed routinely, but can be included for convenience.
6. A second dose of MMR is recommended, at least 1 month after the first dose given. For convenience, options include giving it with the next scheduled vaccination at 18 months of age or with school entry (4-6 years) vaccinations (depending on the provincial/territorial policy), or at any intervening age that is practicable.
7. Delay until subsequent visit if child is < 12 months of age.
8. Recommended schedule and number of doses depend on the product used and the age of the child when vaccination is begun (see page 80 for specific recom-mendations). Not required past age 5.
9. Omit these doses if the previous doses of DTaP and polio were given after the fourth birthday.

National Guidelines for Childhood Immunization Practices

Preamble

The current edition of the Guide contains many examples of the effectiveness of provincial/territorial childhood immunization programs in Canada as carried out by both private and public providers. These include elimination of wild-type poliovirus and a decrease of over 95% in the incidence of *Haemophilus influenzae* type b and measles infections. To ensure continued success it is essential that policy makers, program administrators and providers work together, proactively, to plan, conduct and regularly review childhood immunization programs. Furthermore, several challenges remain, such as continued documented occurrences of "missed opportunities for immunization"; subgroups of Canadian children with lower than optimal vaccine coverage; evidence of incorrect handling and storage of vaccine by providers; wide variations in the reporting of vaccine-associated adverse events; and evidence that there is insufficient communication regarding the risks and benefits of vaccines.

Accordingly, in 1995 the National Advisory Committee on Immunization initiated a process to develop guidelines for childhood immunization practices applicable to both public and private systems of vaccine delivery. The guidelines that follow resulted from extensive consultation, over a 2-year period, with provincial/territorial health authorities; medical, nursing, public health and hospital organizations; and individual providers and child advocacy groups. The guidelines have been officially endorsed by the Canadian Paediatric Society, Advisory Committee on Epidemiology, College of Family Physicians of Canada, Canadian Medical Association, Canadian Nurses Association, Aboriginal Nurses Association of Canada, Society of Obstetricians and Gynaecologists of Canada and the Canadian Public Health Association.

The guidelines are deliberately broad, far-reaching and rigorous. They define the most desirable immunization practices that health care providers can use to assess their own current practices, and identify areas of excellence as well as deficiency. It is recognized that some of the guidelines require involvement of the provinces and territories (e.g., regarding the need to track immunizations and audit coverage levels). Furthermore, some providers/programs may not have the funds necessary to fully implement the guidelines immediately. In such cases the guidelines can act as a tool to clarify immunization needs and to facilitate obtaining additional resources in order to achieve national goals and targets.

The following terms have been used throughout:

- *Provider:* any individual, nurse or physician qualified to give a vaccine

- *Regular provider:* individual usually responsible for a given child's vaccinations

- *Child/children:* the individuals (infancy to adolescence) being considered for immunization

- *Parent:* the individual(s) legally responsible for the child

These guidelines are recommended for use by all health professionals in the public and private sector who administer vaccines to or manage immunization services for infants and children. Although some guidelines will be more directly applicable to one or other setting, all providers and local health officials should collaborate in their efforts to ensure high coverage rates throughout the community and thus achieve and maintain the highest possible degree of community protection against vaccine-preventable diseases.

Guideline 1
Immunization services should be readily available.
Immunization services should be responsive to the needs of parents and children. When feasible, providers should schedule immunization appointments in conjunction with appointments for other health services for children. Immunization services, whether public-health clinics or physicians' offices, should be available during the week and at hours that are convenient for working parents. Services should be available on working days, as well as during some other hours (e.g., weekends, evenings, early mornings, or lunch hours).

Guideline 2
There should be no barriers or unnecessary prerequisites to the receipt of vaccines.
While appointment systems facilitate clinic planning and avoid unnecessarily long waits for children, appointment only systems may act as barriers to the receipt of vaccines. Children who appear on an unscheduled basis for vaccination should be accommodated when possible. Such children should be rapidly and efficiently screened without requiring other comprehensive health services.

A reliable decision to vaccinate can be based exclusively on the information elicited from a parent, and on the provider's observations and judgment about the child's wellness at the time. At a minimum, this includes

- asking the parent if the child is well

- questioning the parent about potential contraindications (Table 2, page 5)

- questioning the parent about reactions to previous vaccinations

- observing the child's general state of health.

Policies and protocols should be developed and implemented so that the administration of vaccine does not depend on individual written orders or on a referral from a primary-care provider.

Guideline 3
Routine childhood immunization services should be publicly funded.
All routine childhood immunizations, as recommended by NACI, should be considered necessary medical services. As such, they should be provided at no charge to patients under provincial and territorial health-service systems.

Guideline 4
Providers should use all clinical encounters to screen for needed vaccines and, when indicated, vaccinate children.
Each encounter with a health-care provider, including those that occur during hospitalization, is an opportunity to review the immunization status, and if indicated, administer needed vaccines. Physicians who offer care to infants and children should consider the immunization status at every visit and offer immunization service as a routine part of that care or encourage attendance at the appropriate public health or physician clinic. At each hospital admission the vaccination record should be reviewed, and before discharge from the hospital, children should receive the vaccines for which they are eligible by age or health status. The child's current immunization provider should be informed about the vaccines administered in hospital. However, successful implementation requires significant improvements in keeping records of immunization histories (see Guideline 9).

Guideline 5
Providers should educate parents in general terms about immunization.
Providers should educate parents in a culturally sensitive way, preferably in their own language, about the importance of vaccination, the diseases vaccines prevent, the recommended immunization schedules, the need to receive vaccines at recommended ages, and the importance of bringing their child's vaccination record to every health-care visit. Parents should be encouraged to take responsibility for ensuring that their child completes the full series. Providers should answer all questions parents may have and provide appropriate education materials at suitable reading levels, preferably in the parents' preferred language. Providers should familiarize themselves with information on immunization provided by the appropriate health departments as well as other sources.

Guideline 6
Providers should inform parents in specific terms about the risks and benefits of vaccines their child is to receive.
Information pamphlets about routine childhood vaccines are available from ministries of health in many provinces and the territories, and also from the Canadian Paediatric Society. Such pamphlets are helpful in answering many questions that parents may

have about immunization. Providers should document in the medical record that they have asked the parents if they have any questions and should ensure that satisfactory answers to any questions were given.

Guideline 7
Providers should recommend deferral or withholding of vaccines for true contraindications only.
There are very few true contraindications to vaccination according to current Canadian guidelines and providers must be aware of them. Accepting conditions that are not true contraindications often results in the needless deferral of indicated vaccines.

Minimal acceptable screening procedures for precautions and contraindications include asking questions to elicit a history of possible adverse events following prior vaccinations, and determining any existing precautions or contraindications (Table 2, page 5).

Guideline 8
Providers should administer all vaccine doses for which a child is eligible at the time of each visit.
Available evidence indicates that most routine childhood vaccines can be administered at the same visit, safely and effectively. Some vaccines are provided in a combination format whereby more than one is given in a single injection and others require separate injection.

Guideline 9
Providers should ensure that all vaccinations are accurately and completely recorded.
9.1 Data to be recorded in the child's record at the time of vaccination
For each vaccine administered the minimum data to be recorded in the child's record should include the name of the vaccine, the date (day, month, and year) and route of administration, the name of the vaccine manufacturer, the lot number, and the name and title of the person administering the vaccine.
9.2 Updating and maintaining the personal vaccination record
All providers should encourage the parents to maintain a copy of their child's personal vaccination record card and present it at each health-care visit so that it can be updated. If a parent fails to bring a child's card, the provider should ensure that adequate information is given so the parent can update the card with the name(s) of the vaccine(s), the date, the provider and the facility.
9.3 Documentation for vaccines given by other providers
Providers should facilitate the transfer of information in the vaccination record to other providers and to appropriate agencies in accordance with legislation.
When a provider who does not routinely vaccinate or care for a child administers a vaccine to that child, the regular provider should be informed.

Guideline 10
Providers should maintain easily retrievable summaries of the vaccination records to facilitate age-appropriate vaccination.

Providers should maintain separate or easily retrievable summaries of vaccination records to facilitate assessment of coverage as well as the identification and recall of children who miss appointments. In addition, immunization files should be sorted periodically, with inactive records placed into a separate file. Providers should indicate in their records, or in an appropriately identified place, all primary-care services that each child receives in order to facilitate scheduling with other services.

Guideline 11
Providers should report clinically significant adverse events following vaccination – promptly, accurately, and completely.

Prompt reporting of adverse events following vaccination is essential to ensure vaccine safety, allowing for timely corrective action when needed, and to continually update information regarding vaccine risk-benefit and contraindications.

Providers should instruct parents to inform them of adverse events following vaccination. Providers should report all clinically significant events to the local public-health authority, regardless of whether they believe the events are caused by the vaccine or not. Providers should fully document the adverse event in the medical record at the time of the event or as soon as possible thereafter. At each immunization visit, information should be sought regarding serious adverse events that may have occurred following previous vaccinations.

Guideline 12
Providers should report all cases of vaccine-preventable diseases as required under provincial and territorial legislation.

Providers should know the local requirements for disease reporting. Reporting of vaccine-preventable diseases is essential for the ongoing evaluation of the effectiveness of immunization programs, to facilitate public-health investigation of vaccine failure, and to facilitate appropriate medical investigation of a child's failure to respond to a vaccine appropriately given.

Guideline 13
Providers should adhere to appropriate procedures for vaccine management.

Vaccines must be handled and stored as recommended in manufacturers' package inserts. The temperatures at which vaccines are transported and stored should be monitored daily. Vaccines must not be administered after their expiry date.

Providers should report usage, wastage, loss, and inventory as required by provincial, territorial or local public-health authorities.

Providers should be familiar with published national and local guidelines for vaccine storage and handling. Providers must ensure that any office staff designated to handle vaccines are also familiar with the guidelines.

Guideline 14
Providers should maintain up-to-date, easily retrievable protocols at all locations where vaccines are administered.
Providers administering vaccines should maintain a protocol that, at a minimum, discusses the appropriate vaccine dosage, vaccine contraindications, the recommended sites and techniques of vaccine administration, as well as possible adverse events and their emergency management. The Canadian Immunization Guide and updates, along with package inserts, can serve as references for the development of protocols. Such protocols should specify the necessary emergency equipment, drugs (including dosage), and personnel to manage safely and competently any medical emergency arising after administration of a vaccine. All providers should be familiar with the content of these protocols, their location, and how to follow them.

Guideline 15
Providers should be properly trained and maintain ongoing education regarding current immunization recommendations.
Vaccines must be administered only by properly trained persons who are recognized as qualified in their specific jurisdiction. Training and ongoing education should be based on current guidelines and recommendations of NACI and provincial and territorial ministries of health, the Guidelines for Childhood Immunization Practices, and other sources of information on immunization.

Guideline 16
Providers should operate a tracking system.
A tracking system should generate reminders of upcoming vaccinations as well as recalls for children who are overdue for their vaccinations. A system may be manual or automated, and may include mailed or telephone messages. All providers should identify, for additional intensive tracking efforts, children considered at high risk for failing to complete the immunization series on schedule (e.g., children who start their series late or children who fall behind schedule).

As an added measure, providers should encourage the development of, and cooperation with, a comprehensive provincial and territorial immunization tracking system.

Guideline 17
Audits should be conducted in all immunization clinics to assess the quality of immunization records and assess immunization coverage levels.
In both public and private sectors, an audit of immunization services should include assessment of all or a random sample of immunization records to assess the quality of documentation, and to determine the immunization coverage level (e.g., the percentage of 2-year-old children who are up-to-date). The results of the audit should be discussed by providers as part of their ongoing quality assurance reviews, and used to develop solutions to the problems identified.

B.   Immunization for Adults

Childhood immunization programs have proven to be an effective and safe method of preventing many infectious diseases. The delivery and implementation of adult immunization programs have not matched the successes achieved in the pediatric population. However, given increased emphasis on disease prevention and health promotion, physicians and the general public must be made aware of the need to improve immunization programs for adults. Immunization status should be considered an integral part of the health assessment of any adult. Opportunities to provide vaccines to adults are being missed.

Prevention of infection by immunization is a lifelong process that should be tailored to meet individual variations in risk resulting from occupation, foreign travel, underlying illness, lifestyle and age. All adults should receive adequate doses of all routinely recommended vaccines, and other vaccinations should be given for selected circumstances when appropriate. Particular emphasis should be placed on improving appropriate utilization of influenza, pneumococcal and hepatitis B vaccines in Canadian adults. For elderly persons, influenza and pneumococcal vaccines are reported as more cost-effective than all other preventive, screening and treatment interventions that have been studied.

Recommended antigens

All Canadian adults require maintenance of immunity to tetanus and diphtheria, preferably with combined (Td) toxoid.

The first priority is to ensure that children receive the recommended series of doses, including the school leaving dose at 14 to 16 years of age, and that adults have completed primary immunization with Td.

The acceptable options for adult booster doses are

1) to continue to offer boosters of Td at 10-yearly intervals at mid decade years, i.e., at age 15, 25, 35, etc. or

2) as a minimum, to review immunization status at least once during adult life, e.g., at 50 years of age, and offer a single dose of Td to everyone who has not had one within the previous 10 years.

In addition, persons who are travelling to areas where they are likely to be exposed to diphtheria may be offered a booster dose of Td if more than 10 years have elapsed since their most recent booster.

Persons ≥ 65 years of age should receive influenza vaccine every year and, on a one-time basis, a dose of pneumococcal vaccine. Special recall strategies may be necessary to ensure high coverage, particularly for those who are at greatest risk of influenza-related complications, e.g., people with chronic cardiopulmonary disease. Adults < 65 with high-risk medical conditions for complications of influenza and pneumococcal infection should also receive influenza vaccine every year and a single dose of pneumococcal vaccine (see pages 105 and 141 for high-risk conditions).

Adults born before 1970 may be considered immune to measles. Adults born in 1970 or later who do not have documentation of adequate measles immunization or who are known to be seronegative should receive measles vaccine (given as MMR). For adults who have already received one dose of measles vaccine, a second dose of vaccine would provide optimal protection. Priority for a second dose should be given to health care workers, college students and travellers to areas where measles is epidemic.

Most individuals born before 1970 may also be considered immune to mumps. Mumps vaccine (given as MMR) is recommended for young adults with no history of mumps.

Rubella vaccine should be given to all female adolescents and women of childbearing age unless they have documented evidence of detectable antibody or documented evidence of vaccination. Combined measles, mumps and rubella (MMR) vaccine is preferred. In addition, MMR vaccine should be given to rubella-susceptible health care workers of either sex who may, through frequent face-to-face contact, expose pregnant women to rubella.

Adults who are at increased risk of exposure to hepatitis B by virtue of their occupation, lifestyle or environment should receive hepatitis B vaccine (see pages 95-96).

In the future, booster doses of adult formulation of acellular pertussis vaccine may be recommended to prevent occurrence and spread of the disease. Further studies are needed in this area.

Table 4 lists antigens that are indicated for routine use in adults. Detailed information on immunization for health care workers and travellers can be found in Part 5 and 6 (pages 187 and 191) of the Guide.

Table 4
Routine Immunization of Adults

Vaccine or toxoid	Indication	Further doses
Diphtheria (adult preparation)	All adults	Every 10 years, preferably given with tetanus toxoid (Td) See pages 74-75
Tetanus	All adults	Every 10 years, preferably given as Td See page 165
Influenza	Adults ≥ 65 years; adults < 65 years at high risk of influenza-related complications	Every year using current vaccine formulation See pages 105-106
Pneumococcal	Adults ≥ 65 years; conditions with increased risk of pneumococcal diseases	None usually, but see page 142
Measles	All adults born in 1970 or later who are susceptible to measles	See page 121, preferably given as MMR
Rubella	Susceptible women of childbearing age and health care workers	None
Mumps	Adults born in 1970 or later with no history of mumps	None

Strategies to improve vaccine delivery to adults

Despite favourable attitudes among Canadian physicians towards the use of vaccines in adults, such vaccines are underused. It is estimated that only 45% of high-risk individuals receive influenza vaccine annually. An organized systematic approach to vaccine delivery is required. Physicians play a major role in the identification of adults in need of immunization. Methods of identification include reminder notices in patient records, pre-employment medical examinations, school and college entry questionnaires, employee health nurse visits and letter reminders. Emergency rooms, public health clinics, hospitals and other health care institutions may also play an important role in vaccine delivery. When persons are offered vaccines, high rates of compliance are usually noted. Adult immunization can be successful if well organized provincial/territorial/institutional programs are established. See Table 5 for a summary of immunization in selected cases.

Teenagers and young adults require special attention. Some may not have received recommended vaccines while others may have received vaccines of lower potency than those currently available. Given the infrequency with which this group seeks medical care, practitioners and health officials should use every opportunity to review and update their protection.

Table 5
Summary of Selected Immunization for Adults

Vaccine	Indication	Further doses if risk continues
BCG	High-risk exposure	None
Hepatitis B	Occupational, life-style or environmental exposure	None
Japanese encephalitis	Travel to endemic area or other exposure risk	See page 114
Meningococcal	High-risk exposure	See pages 126-128
Pertussis	Not indicated	
Poliomyelitis	Travel to endemic area or other exposure risk	See pages 147 and 192
Rabies pre-exposure use	Occupational or other risk	Every 2 years, see page 155
Typhoid	High-risk exposure	Every 3-4 years, see pages 170-171
Yellow fever	Travel to endemic area or if required for foreign travel	Every 10 years, see page 176

Part 2 – Recommended Immunization for Infants, Children and Adults

C.   Opportunity for Immunization in Acute Care Institutions/Facilities

A vaccination history taken on admission to hospital provides an important opportunity to ensure that up-to-date immunization is maintained in all individuals.

In acute care hospitals, the admission of elderly individuals and others at high risk of influenza-related complications, especially those with chronic cardiopulmonary disease, should be regarded as an opportunity to ensure their protection against influenza. Programs to immunize such patients prior to discharge are an effective means of ensuring that they receive vaccines.

Pneumococcal vaccine should be administered prior to discharge to previously unvaccinated (eligible) patients > 65 years of age and those with a significant condition for which vaccine is recommended.

All pregnant women should be screened for hepatitis B surface antigen (HBsAg), and the newborn of an HBsAg positive woman should be given hepatitis B immune globulin (HBIG) and started on a course of HB vaccine.

Susceptible women should receive rubella vaccine in the immediate post-partum period before discharge from hospital.

D. Immunization of Persons in Long-Term Health Care Facilities

It is important to ensure that children living in chronic care institutions receive all routine vaccinations for their age. Adults should be immunized against tetanus and diphtheria. If required, a primary series should be administered, although in most cases only a booster dose(s), repeated every 10 years, will be needed.

Annual vaccination against influenza is strongly recommended for individuals in nursing homes and chronic care institutions. A program to ensure annual influenza vaccination should be in place.

Pneumococcal vaccine is recommended for the elderly and the chronically ill, particularly in closed populations. A single dose of the vaccine should be administered to all previously unvaccinated individuals admitted to such facilities.

Individuals in institutions for the developmentally challenged should receive both hepatitis A and B vaccines.

SELECTED REFERENCES

ACP Task Force on Adult Immunization and Infectious Diseases Society of America. *Guide for adult immunization*. 2nd ed. Philadelphia, PA: American College of Physicians, 1990.

American Academy of Pediatrics. Committee on Infectious Diseases. *Immunization of adolescents: recommendations of the Advisory Committee on Immigration Practices, the American Academy of Pediatrics, the American Academy of Family Physicians, and the American Medical Association.* Pediatrics 1997;99:479-88.

CDC. National Immunization Program. *Adult immunization : a report by the National Vaccine Advisory Committee, National Vaccine Program.* Atlanta, GA: U.S. Department of Health & Human Services, 1994.

CDC. *Update on adult immunization: recommendations of the Advisory Committee on Immunization Practices(ACIP).* MMWR 1991;40(No. RR-12):1-94.

Gardner P, Schaffner W. *Immunization of adults*. N Engl J Med 1993;328;1252-58.

Williams WW, Hickson MA, Kane MA et al. *Immunization policies and vaccine coverage among adults: the risk for missed opportunities.* Ann Intern Med 1988;108;616-25.

Part 3
ACTIVE IMMUNIZING AGENTS

BCG VACCINE

Mortality and morbidity from tuberculosis (TB) have declined significantly in Canada since the Second World War (Figure 1). There was a 30% decrease in the number of reported cases of TB from 1980 (2,762 cases) to 1995 (1,930 cases). Since 1988 approximately 2,000 cases have been reported annually. The reported incidence of cases among children < 5 years was 4.6/100,000 in 1995.

Figure 1: Tuberculosis - Reported Cases, 1924-1995 and Deaths, 1937-1994, Canada

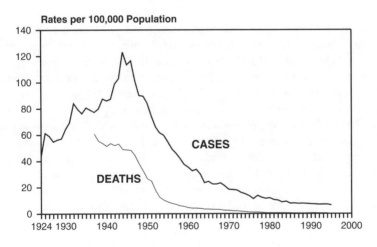

Among infectious diseases, TB is a leading cause of morbidity and mortality worldwide. There is growing global concern about the emergence of drug-resistant strains, which are threatening to make TB incurable again; moreover, the resurgence of the disease is being accelerated by the spread of human immunodeficiency virus (HIV). In 1993, the WHO declared tuberculosis to be a "global emergency".

BCG Vaccine

In Canada, the incidence of TB varies from one geographic region to another. Rates increase with age among both sexes, particularly among males. Groups at highest risk include Native populations and immigrants from areas with a high prevalence of the disease. Other persons at high risk include those infected with both HIV and tubercle bacilli, close contacts of persons with untreated TB, the elderly and the homeless.

TB control measures include 1) early identification of persons with active (infectious) disease and treatment of each case until cured; 2) appropriate use of preventive chemotherapy for persons infected with *Mycobacterium tuberculosis* but without active disease; 3) measures in health care facilities and other institutions to prevent nosocomial/institutional spread; and 4) BCG vaccination of selected population groups.

Preparations Used for Immunization

Bacille Calmette-Guérin (BCG) vaccine contains live attenuated bacteria of a strain of *M. bovis*. It is available as a lyophilized preparation for intradermal/intracutaneous use. Instructions in the manufacturer's product leaflet should always be followed for suspending and administering vaccine, especially when BCG vaccine is used in children < 2 years, since the dose is reduced.

There are many BCG vaccines available in the world today. All are derived from the original strain, but they vary in immunogenicity, efficacy and reactogenicity. In particular, the field efficacy of BCG immunization has varied in several studies. A recent meta-analysis of 13 prospective studies showed an overall protective effect of 51% (95% confidence interval 30%-66%) in preventing TB and a 71% (95% confidence interval 47%-84%) protective effect against death due to tuberculosis. An analysis of 10 case-control studies showed similar results, with a protective effect of 50% (95% confidence interval 36%-61%) against TB. The protective effect was greater among infants and children than adults in the meta-analyses. An enhanced protective effect was also noted in studies in which BCG was given to newborns or infants. These studies are consistent with two case-control studies involving Canadian Aboriginal populations. Five studies reporting on tuberculous meningitis showed a protective effect of 64% (95% confidence interval 30%-82%).

The protective effect of vaccination increases with increased distance from the equator. The significance of this finding is unclear at present. Many factors have been considered to explain variations among studies, including BCG strain, infection with non-tuberculous mycobacteria, climate, storage of vaccine, vitamin D and sunlight, and population genetics. BCG strain differences were not an independent risk factor in the meta-analysis. At the present time there is no clear explanation for the variation among studies or in the duration of immunity where efficacy has been shown.

BCG Vaccine

The BCG vaccines available in Canada are licensed for their ability to produce a positive tuberculin reaction. In individuals receiving BCG immunization to prevent TB a positive tuberculin skin test usually results. However, there is no clear relationship between the development of cutaneous delayed type hypersensitivity and protection from tuberculous disease.

Storage requirements
The vaccine should be protected from heat and direct sunlight and stored according to the manufacturer's instructions, usually at a temperature not greater than 5° C. Reconstituted freeze-dried vaccine should be kept refrigerated when not in use and discarded if not used within 8 hours.

Preparations Used for Immunotherapy
Lyophilized preparations of BCG for intravesical use in the treatment of primary and relapsed carcinoma *in situ* of the urinary bladder are formulated at a much higher strength and must **not** be used for TB immunization purposes.

Recommended Usage
Because BCG vaccination usually results in a positive tuberculin skin test, the benefits gained by BCG vaccination must be carefully weighed against the potential loss of the tuberculin test as a primary tool to identify infection with *M. tuberculosis*. In Canada, TB rates are relatively low, and the tuberculin test has become increasingly useful as an epidemiologic, case finding and diagnostic tool. In the United States, the increase in rates of multidrug-resistant TB has led to a re-evaluation of the use of BCG in selected settings as a primary intervention, but no broadening of criteria for more widespread use has been suggested.

BCG should be given only to persons with a negative tuberculin skin test (Mantoux 5 TU PPD-S). Infants < 6 weeks of age do not need to be tuberculin tested before receiving BCG vaccine since reactivity does not develop before this age.

BCG immunization will not prevent the development of active TB in individuals who are already infected with *M. tuberculosis*.

BCG vaccine is recommended for the following persons:

1. Infants and children belonging to groups experiencing a high rate of new infections, i.e., in excess of 1% per year, when other control measures have proved ineffective.

2. Infants and children with negative tuberculin skin tests who are 1) at high risk of intimate and prolonged exposure to persistently untreated or ineffectively treated patients with infectious pulmonary TB and who cannot be removed from the source of exposure or be placed on long-term preventive therapy, or are 2) continuously exposed to persons with TB who have bacilli resistant to isoniazid and rifampin.

3. Individuals repeatedly exposed to persons with untreated or inadequately treated active TB in conditions under which normal preventive measures are not possible or have been unsuccessful, e.g., when multidrug-resistant TB is involved.

4. BCG vaccination may be considered for health care workers (including medical laboratory workers) at considerable risk of exposure to tubercle bacilli, especially drug-resistant bacilli, in situations in which protective measures against infection are known to be ineffective or not feasible. Consultation with a regional TB and/or infectious disease expert is recommended prior to administering BCG vaccine.

5. BCG vaccination may be considered for travellers planning extended stays in areas of high tuberculosis prevalence, particularly where a program of serial skin testing and appropriate chemoprophylaxis may not be feasible or where primary isoniazid resistance of *Mycobacterium tuberculosis* is high. Travellers are advised to consult a specialist in travel medicine or infectious disease when considering a decision for or against BCG immunization.

Usual Response to Vaccination

The development of erythema, papule formation or superficial ulceration 3 to 6 weeks after intradermal BCG injection usually indicates successful vaccination. Some enlargement of the regional lymph nodes usually accompanies the lesions at the vaccination site. Most authorities believe that development of a typical pustule and scar at the vaccination site indicates that protection has been conferred.

The relationship of the development of a positive tuberculin skin test with the protective efficacy of BCG has not been well studied. However, present methods of vaccination usually induce positive tuberculin tests for approximately 5 years in the majority of vaccinees. The size of response to a tuberculin skin test decreases with time. Tuberculin reactivity may be diminished or transiently abolished during the course of certain viral infections, particularly measles.

Revaccination with BCG is not recommended and should be addressed in consultation with regional TB or infectious disease experts. Tuberculin skin testing used as a basis for decisions on BCG revaccination should be discontinued.

Adverse Reactions

Adverse reactions are more common in young vaccinees (infants vs older children) and are frequently related to improper technique in administration (mainly improper dilution). Most reactions are generally mild and do not require treatment. The current infant dose of vaccine has decreased the incidence of these reactions among infants to less than 2%.

Common reactions include persistent or spreading skin ulceration at the vaccination site, inflammatory adenitis and keloid formation. Moderately severe and, very rarely, severe reactions can occur. Rates of such incidents appear to vary with the strain of vaccine, dose and method of vaccination and the age of the recipient. Moderately severe reactions, such as marked lymphadenitis or suppurative adenitis, occur in 0.2 to 4.0 per 1,000 vaccinees.

Disseminated BCG infection, which may be fatal, occurs very rarely (about 1 in 1 million vaccinations), and is seen almost exclusively in persons with impaired immune responses. Three such cases (two fatal) in severely immunocompromised infants have been reported in Canada between 1993 and 1998. One was associated with HIV infection. Severe osteitis/osteomyelitis can also occur very rarely.

Contraindications (Table 1)

BCG vaccination is contraindicated for persons with immune deficiency diseases including HIV infection, altered immune status due to malignant disease, and impaired

Table 1
Precautions/Contraindications in BCG Vaccination

	NACI	BCG-1*	BCG-2†
Should not be given with another (live virus) vaccine	X	X	X
DPT 15 days before or after		X	
Sufficient time before to let reaction subside or after to let BCG reaction subside			X
One month must elapse after the injection of viral vaccines before giving BCG	X	X	
Should not be given within 4 weeks of administration of a measles (live virus) containing vaccine	X		
Not recommended in pregnancy	X	X	X
Immunosuppression	X	X	X
Burns/extensive active skin disease	X		X
Febrile symptoms or other signs of acute illness		X	

* BCG-1 BioVax
† BCG-2 Pasteur Mérieux Connaught Canada

BCG Vaccine

immune function secondary to treatment with corticosteroids, chemotherapeutic agents or radiation. Extensive skin disease or burns is also a contraindication. BCG is contraindicated for individuals with a positive tuberculin skin test, although vaccination of tuberculin reactors has frequently occurred without incident.

BCG should not be given within 4 weeks after administration of any live vaccine, since these vaccines are known to suppress the tuberculin reaction.

Vaccination of pregnant women should preferably be delayed until after delivery, although no harmful effects on the fetus have been observed.

The vaccine should not be administered to individuals receiving drugs with antituberculous activity since these agents may be active against the vaccine strain.

Other Considerations

BCG vaccine does not provide permanent or absolute protection against TB. This disease should be considered as a possible diagnosis in any vaccinee who presents with suggestive history, signs or symptoms of TB.

Past history of BCG vaccination should not preclude tuberculin skin testing in BCG vaccinees exposed to an individual with active TB. Refer to the *Canadian tuberculosis standards* for assistance in the interpretation of tuberculin skin tests in exposed individuals who are immunocompetent, immunodeficient or have a history of BCG vaccination. Caution should be used when attributing tuberculin positivity to BCG vaccination, since it is not possible to absolutely differentiate between a positive tuberculin test due to BCG and one resulting from TB infection.

Interpretation of the PPD test result in BCG-vaccinated groups should ignore the history of BCG status when contacts of active cases are being investigated. If BCG was received in infancy, it can be ignored in all population groups. If BCG was received after infancy, it can be considered the cause of a significant test reaction if the expected prevalence of TB infection in the population is lower than 10% (i.e., in the general population of non-Aboriginal Canadians or in immigrants from industrialized countries). BCG given after infancy can be ignored as a cause of tuberculin reactions among immigrants from countries with high rates of tuberculosis or among those who are at high risk for tuberculosis, such as contacts of an active case, patients with abnormal x-ray or with HIV infection, or Aboriginal Canadians.

BCG Vaccine

SELECTED REFERENCES

Brewer TF, Colditz GA. *Relationship between bacille Calmette-Guérin (BCG) strains and the efficacy of BCG vaccine in the prevention of tuberculosis.* Clin Infect Dis 1995;20:126-35.

Canadian Lung Association. *Canadian tuberculosis standards.* Ottawa, 1996.

Ciesielski SD. *BCG vaccination and the PPD test: what the clinician needs to know.* J Fam Pract 1995;40:76-80.

Colditz GA, Berkey CS, Mosteller et al. *The efficacy of Bacillus Calmette-Guérin vaccination of newborns in the prevention of tuberculosis: meta-analyses of the published literature.* Pediatrics 1995;96:29-35.

Colditz GA, Brewer TF, Berkey CS et al. *Efficacy of BCG vaccine in the prevention of tuberculosis.* JAMA 1994;271:698-702.

Fine PE. *Bacille Calmette-Guérin vaccines: a rough guide.* Clin Infect Dis 1995;20:11-4.

Global tuberculosis programme and global programme on vaccines. Statement on BCG revaccination for the prevention of tuberculosis. Wkly Epidemiol Rec 1995;70:229-31.

Houston S, Fanning A, Soskoline C et al. *The effectiveness of bacillus Calmette-Guérin (BCG) vaccination against tuberculosis: a case-control study in treaty Indians, Alberta, Canada.* Am J Epidemiol 1990;131:340-48.

Lotte A, Wasz-Hockert O, Poisson N et al. *BCG complications.* Adv Tuberc Res 1984;21;107-93.

O'Brien KL, Ruff AJ, Louis MA et al. *Bacille Calmette-Guérin complications in children born to HIV-1 infected women with a review of the literature.* Pediatrics 1995;95:414-18.

Pabst HF, Godel J, Grace M et al. *Effect of breast-feeding on immune response to BCG vaccination.* Lancet 1989;1:295-97.

Roche PW, Triccas JA, Winter N. *BCG vaccination against tuberculosis: past disappointments and future hopes.* Trends Microbiol 1995;3:397-401.

Watson JM. *BCG — mass or selective vaccination?* J Hosp Infect 1995;30 (June suppl):508-13.

BCG Vaccine

CHOLERA VACCINE

Cholera is an acute bacterial infection that presents as profuse, watery diarrhea. It is associated with rapid dehydration and occasionally hypovolemic shock, which may be life-threatening. The disease is caused by an enterotoxin produced by *Vibrio cholerae*. Two serogroups, 01 and 0139 (Bengal), have been implicated in human epidemics. Within the serogroup 01 are the classical and El Tor biotypes.

Mortality ranges from over 50% without treatment to less than 1% among adequately treated patients. Treatment consists mainly of either oral or parenteral rehydration. Infection is generally acquired from contaminated water or food, particularly undercooked or raw shellfish and fish. The ratio of symptomatic to asymptomatic (carrier) cases varies from strain to strain. In El Tor infections, the ratio of symptomatic to asymptomatic cases (1:50) is much lower than in cholera infection due to the classical biotype (1:5). Humans are the only known natural host.

The seventh pandemic began in 1961 with *V. cholerae* of the El Tor biotype spreading through southern Asia, the Middle East, Eastern Europe and, in 1970, Africa. In 1991, the El Tor biotype caused an outbreak in Peru, which led to an extensive epidemic in other Amazonian and Central American countries. In Canada, between 1993 and 1996 there were 23 reported cases of the biotype El Tor or Ogawa. Travel history was not reported for all cases, but from the information available, the destinations included El Salvador, Mexico, the Dominican Republic, India and Pakistan. Many of these people had travelled to private homes. No secondary transmission was noted. In countries with modern sanitation, good hygiene and clean water supplies, the risk of transmission is low. For travellers, prevention relies on care in the choice of food and water supply and in using good hygienic measures rather than on vaccination.

Preparations Used for Immunization

Parenteral, inactivated cholera vaccine offers short, limited effectiveness and is not recommended for Canadians travelling to endemic areas.

Oral, live attenuated cholera vaccine (CVD 103-HgR) has recently been licensed in Canada. The vaccine also contains aspartame (a phenylalanine derivative), which is added as a sweetener. The buffer solution contains sodium bicarbonate, ascorbic acid and lactose, which serve to neutralize gastric acid.

Seroconversion rates over 90% have been reported after a single oral dose of the vaccine. Seroconversion occurred as early as 8 days after administration of the vaccine and lasted for 6 months.

The protective efficacy of the vaccine has been tested in volunteers challenged with pathogenic *Vibrio cholerae* of both biotypes and serotypes. Protection against the classic biotype was demonstrated among 82% to 100% of subjects, and against the El Tor biotype among 62% to 67% of subjects exposed.

There is no cholera vaccine currently available that has been shown to protect against the 0139 Bengal strain in South Asia.

The oral cholera vaccine (CVD 103-HgR) has not been shown to offer protection against enterotoxigenic *Escherichia coli* (ETEC)-associated diarrhea, which is a common cause of diarrhea in travellers.

An experimental oral vaccine containing cholera toxin B-subunit and whole inactivated cholera bacteria (BS-WC), which is not currently licensed in Canada (as of 1997), may offer some protection against ETEC-associated diarrhea as well as against cholera.

Storage requirements
Oral cholera vaccine (CVD 103-HgR) should be stored between 2° and 8° C and should not be frozen. The reconstituted vaccine should be ingested as soon after mixing as possible.

Recommended Usage
Travellers should take all the necessary precautions to avoid contact with or ingestion of potentially contaminated food or water since not all recipients of the vaccine will be fully protected against cholera.

The World Health Organization indicates that since 1992 no country or territory has required a certificate of vaccination against cholera. Cholera vaccine is no longer required or recommended for the vast majority of Canadian travellers. Persons following the usual tourist itineraries in countries affected by cholera are at virtually no risk of acquiring infection. Travellers who may be at increased risk for acquiring cholera (e.g., health professionals working in endemic areas or workers in refugee camps) may benefit from vaccination. A detailed, individual risk assessment should be made in order to determine which travellers may benefit from vaccination.

Oral cholera vaccine is given in a single dose as a drink mixed with the provided buffer solution in cold or luke warm water. It is approved for adults and children > 2 years. It should be given 1 hour before food or drink.

An optimal booster dose or interval has not yet been established. However, the manufacturer recommends that a repeat dose be given as described every 6 months, if indicated.

Adverse Reactions

Adverse reactions to oral cholera vaccine have been mild in nature and of short duration. Reported adverse reactions include nausea, abdominal cramps and diarrhea. The side-effect profile was similar for placebo recipients.

Contraindications and Precautions

Hypersensitivity to the vaccine or the buffer components is a contraindication to further doses. Since the vaccine is a live one it should be used with caution in immunocompromised or immunosuppressed individuals, or pregnant women. A risk/benefit analysis should be used to determine whether an individual in these groups should be immunized. Excretion of vaccine organisms is minimal, and spread to contacts of vaccinated persons is unlikely. The vaccine should not be given during an acute febrile illness or to any person with acute gastrointestinal disease.

Antibiotics may interfere with the effectiveness of the vaccine. Persons receiving therapy with antibiotics should wait 7 days after the completion of therapy before taking the oral cholera vaccine.

Antimalarial prophylaxis may also interfere with the effectiveness of the vaccine and therefore antimalarial prophylaxis should start no sooner than 7 days after administration of the oral cholera vaccine.

The concomitant administration of oral polio vaccine or yellow fever vaccine does not interfere with the immune response to oral cholera vaccine.

The administration of oral typhoid vaccine (Ty21a) and oral cholera vaccine should be separated by at least 8 hours.

SELECTED REFERENCES

Committee to Advise on Tropical Medicine and Travel and the National Advisory Committee on Immunization. *Preliminary conjoint statement on oral cholera vaccination.* CCDR 1996;22:73-5.

Cyrz SJ, Levine MM, Kaper JB et al. *Randomized, double-blind, placebo-controlled trial to evaluate the safety and immunogenicity of the live cholera vaccine strain CVD-HgR in Swiss adults.* Vaccine 1990;8:577-80.

Kotloff KL, Wasserman SS, O'Donnell S et al. *Safety and immunogenicity in North Americans of a single dose of live oral cholera vaccine CVD 103-HgR: results of a placebo-controlled, double-blind crossover trial.* Infect Immun 1992;60:4430-32.

MacPherson DW, Tonkin M. *Cholera vaccination: a decision analysis.* Can Med Assoc J 1992;146:1947-52.

Peltola H, Siitonen A, Kyronseppa H et al. *Prevention of traveller's diarrhea by oral B-subunit/whole-cell cholera vaccine.* Lancet 1991;338:1285-89.

Cholera Vaccine

DIPHTHERIA TOXOID

Diphtheria is a serious communicable disease caused by toxigenic strains of *Corynebacterium diphtheriae*. The case-fatality rate remains 5% to 10%, with highest death rates in the very young and the elderly. The organism may be harboured in the nasopharynx, skin and other sites of asymptomatic carriers, making eradication of the disease difficult.

Routine immunization against diphtheria in infancy and childhood has been widely practised in Canada since 1930. In 1924, 9,000 cases were reported, the highest recorded annual incidence in Canada (Figure 1). At the same time diphtheria was one of the most common causes of death in children from 1 to 5 years of age. By the mid-1950s, routine immunization had resulted in a remarkable decline in the morbidity and mortality of the disease. Since the early 1980s, diphtheria incidence has remained at extremely low levels, with only 2 to 5 cases reported annually from 1986 to 1995 (the majority in persons aged ≥ 20 years who lacked protection) and no cases reported in 1996. No deaths have been reported since 1983.

Figure 1: Diphtheria - Reported Cases, Canada, 1924-1996

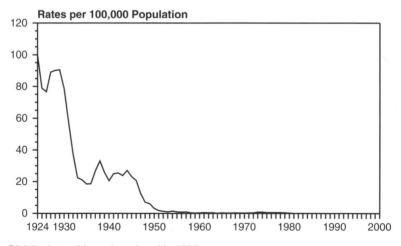

Diphtheria toxoid was introduced in 1926.

Toxigenic strains of diphtheria bacilli are still detected each year in carriers (pharyngeal, skin and ear), sometimes associated with mild clinical symptoms. Asymptomatic carriage of *C. diphtheriae* is far more common than clinical diphtheria. The disease occurs most frequently in unimmunized or partially immunized individuals. Although occasional cases of mild clinical diphtheria do occur in apparently fully immunized persons, antitoxin stimulated by immunization is believed to persist at protective levels for 10 years or more. Recent serosurveys of healthy adult populations in Canada indicate that approximately 20% of those surveyed (higher in some age groups) do not have protective levels of antibody to diphtheria. The actual levels of serosusceptibility in the general adult population may be even higher. The potential for disease re-emergence if immunization levels are allowed to fall and adults do not receive booster doses has been demonstrated most recently in the Commonwealth of Independent States (former Soviet Union), where tens of thousands of cases with substantial mortality have been reported.

Preparations Used for Immunization

Diphtheria toxoid is a cell-free preparation of diphtheria toxin detoxified with formaldehyde. It is highly immunogenic, but two to three primary doses are necessary to ensure reliable seroconversion and sufficiently high concentrations of protective antibody. Titres decline slowly with time but can be boosted by additional doses. The significance for protection against diphtheria of loss of antitoxin in adequately immunized persons is not clear. The immunity conferred is antitoxic, not antibacterial, and thus protects against the potentially lethal systemic effects of diphtheria toxin but not directly against local infection. However, carriage of *C. diphtheriae* has been observed to be lower in immunized populations.

Diphtheria toxoid is available as a preparation adsorbed with aluminum phosphate and combined with other toxoids or vaccines (e.g., tetanus, poliomyelitis or pertussis, see Appendix III). The amount of toxoid present is measured in flocculating units (Lf). It should be noted that the amount of diphtheria toxoid in combined preparations of diphtheria and tetanus toxoids varies widely with the product and manufacturer. Preparations containing only 2 Lf of diphtheria toxoid (commonly designated Td) are intended for use in persons ≥ 7 years of age.

Recommended Usage

Routine immunization against diphtheria is recommended for all persons regardless of age at which immunization is begun. Adsorbed vaccines must be injected intramuscularly.

Primary immunization of children < 7 years of age

It is preferable to use products in which diphtheria toxoid is combined with pertussis vaccine and tetanus toxoid (DPT) or with tetanus toxoid and acellular pertussis vaccine (DTaP), with or without inactivated poliomyelitis vaccine (DPT-polio or DTaP-polio) and *Haemophilus influenzae* type b conjugate vaccine. The primary immunizing course of diphtheria toxoid alone or in combination consists of four doses and should ideally begin at 2 months of age (see Part 2: Recommended Immunization Schedules). The recommended time interval between the initial three doses is normally 8 weeks (but should not be less than 4 weeks); the fourth dose should be given 6 to 12 months after the third dose. A booster dose is recommended 30 to 54 months after the fourth dose, most commonly at 4 to 6 years (school entry). This booster dose is not necessary if the fourth dose in the primary series was given on or after the fourth birthday. Although diphtheria toxoid is not required in this case, a fifth dose of pertussis vaccine is strongly recommended and is most easily given combined with diphtheria and tetanus toxoids. An additional booster dose of adult-type preparation (Td) should be given at 14 to 16 years of age (school leaving booster) and at least once again during adult life (see below).

Primary immunization of persons ≥ 7 years of age

The recommended agent is a combined adsorbed tetanus and diphtheria preparation (Td, adult-type) containing less diphtheria toxoid than preparations given to younger children. This is less likely to cause reactions in older persons. Two doses are given 4 to 8 weeks apart, with a further dose 6 to 12 months later to complete the course.

Booster doses

The need for *regular boosters* during adult life has never been established. In Canada and the U.S., diphtheria rarely develops in adults who have completed a primary series of vaccinations, despite a general failure to observe the recommendation for 10-yearly boosters. At the same time, the contribution of limited compliance with this recommendation to the current favourable disease control status is unknown. Consequently, there are few firm data on which to base a recommendation for less frequent boosters, and it is known that antitoxin levels decline with time.

Ensuring that children receive the recommended series of doses, *including the school leaving dose* at 14 to 16 years of age, and that adults have completed primary immunization should be the first priority.

The acceptable options for adult booster doses are:

■ to continue to offer boosters of Td at 10-yearly intervals or

■ as a minimum, to review immunization status at least once during adult life, e.g., at 50 years of age, and offer a single dose of Td to everyone who has not had one within the previous 10 years.

In addition,

- Persons who are travelling to areas where they are likely to be exposed to diphtheria may be offered a booster dose of Td if more than 10 years have elapsed since their most recent booster.

- If a case of diphtheria occurs, close contacts (household, classroom or similar) should be given a dose of a toxoid preparation appropriate to their age unless they are known to be fully immunized, with the last dose given in the previous 10 years. The remaining doses required to provide full immunization should be given to any contacts who were previously unimmunized or incompletely immunized. Patients convalescent from diphtheria should be given a complete primary course of toxoid, unless serologic testing indicates protective levels of antitoxin, since diphtheria infection does not always confer immunity.

Persons requiring a booster dose of tetanus toxoid for wound management should receive Td as a convenient means of reinforcing their diphtheria protection.

Adverse Reactions

Diphtheria toxoid may cause severe but transient local and febrile reactions in children and adults, the frequency increasing with age, the dose of toxoid and the number of doses given. In up to 70% of children receiving a booster dose of currently used adsorbed DPT vaccine at 4 to 6 years of age, local redness and/or swelling of 5 cm or more in diameter have been reported. When a booster dose of Td is given at 14 to 16 years of age, only 10% experience marked local reactions.

Contraindications and Precautions

Persons ≥ 7 years of age should only be given preparations formulated for older children and adults. Before giving a combined vaccine, it is most important to ensure that there are no contraindications to the administration of any of the other components.

When a combined diphtheria-tetanus preparation is being considered, care should be taken to avoid administration of tetanus toxoid more frequently than is recommended (see section on Tetanus Toxoid) or adverse reactions may result.

Care should be taken to ensure that adsorbed products are given intramuscularly, since subcutaneous injection of adsorbed products produces a much higher rate of local reactions.

Combined Vaccines against Diphtheria, Pertussis, Tetanus and Poliomyelitis

It is recommended that diphtheria and tetanus toxoids, and pertussis and poliomyelitis vaccines be administered in a combined formulation with either whole-cell or acellular pertussis vaccine.

Diphtheria Toxoid

Adsorbed vaccines must be administered intramuscularly, in accordance with the manufacturer's instructions, to minimize the degree of local reaction.

Local and systemic reactions associated in the past with the primary series of DPT or DPT-polio containing whole-cell pertussis vaccine appear to have been due primarily to the pertussis component. Reaction rates of the combined vaccines were similar to those of pertussis vaccine alone. Vaccines containing acellular pertussis vaccine have much lower rates of adverse reaction, but local reactions may be observed with the fourth and fifth doses of vaccine.

A combined adsorbed product containing diphtheria and tetanus toxoids and inactivated poliomyelitis vaccine is available for children < 7 years of age in whom pertussis vaccine is contraindicated.

Combined adsorbed preparations of diphtheria and tetanus toxoid formulated for adults (Td) are the preferred immunizing agents for persons ≥ 7 years of age. They are recommended in the following cases:

1. primary immunization of older children and adults against diphtheria and tetanus;

2. regular booster doses for children at 14 to 16 years of age, and for adults;

3. management of wounds when tetanus toxoid is indicated.

A combined adsorbed preparation containing diphtheria and tetanus toxoids, and inactivated poliomyelitis vaccine (Td-polio) is available for immunization of older children ≥ 7 years and selected adults. For details of usage and precautions to be taken, see relevant sections of the Guide.

Discussion of control of cases and outbreaks in the community are beyond the scope of this Guide. Guidelines by the Advisory Committee on Epidemiology on the control of diphtheria in the community will be published in the near future in the Canada Communicable Disease Report.

SELECTED REFERENCES

Galazka AM, Robertson SE. *Immunization against diphtheria with special emphasis on immunization of adults.* Vaccine 1996;14:845-57.

Galazka AM, Robertson SE, Oblapenko GP. *Resurgence of diphtheria.* Eur J Epidemiol 1995;11:95-105.

Gupta RK, Griffin Jr. P, Xu J et al. *Diphtheria antitoxin levels in US blood and plasma donors.* J Infect Dis 1996;173:1493-97.

Larsen K, Ullberg-Olsson K, Ekwall E et al. *The immunization of adults against diphtheria in Sweden.* J Biol Stand 1987;15:109-16.

Maple PA, Efstratiou A, George RC et al. *Diphtheria immunity in UK blood donors.* Lancet 1995;345:963-65.

Simonsen O, Kjeldsen K, Vendborg H-A et al. *Revaccination of adults against diphtheria 1: responses and reactions to different doses of diphtheria toxoid in 30-70-years-old persons with low serum antitoxin levels.* Acta Path Microbiol Immunol Scand Sect C 1986;94:213-18.

Yuan L, Lau W, Thipphawong J et al. *Diphtheria and tetanus immunity among blood donors in Toronto.* Can Med Assoc J 1997;156:985-90.

Diphtheria Toxoid

HAEMOPHILUS VACCINE

Haemophilus influenzae type b (Hib) was the most common cause of bacterial meningitis and a leading cause of other serious invasive infections in young children prior to the introduction of Hib vaccines. About 55% to 65% of affected children had meningitis while the remainder had epiglottitis, bacteremia, cellulitis, pneumonia or septic arthritis. The case-fatality rate of meningitis is about 5%. Severe neurologic sequelae occur in 10% to 15% of survivors and deafness in 15% to 20% (severe in 3% to 7%).

Before the introduction of Hib conjugate vaccines in Canada in 1988, there were approximately 2,000 cases of Hib disease annually. Since then the overall incidence has fallen by more than 90%. The majority of cases occur now in children too old to have received primary vaccination. In 1996, only 26 cases were reported in children < 5 years of age.

H. Influenzae is also commonly associated with otitis media, sinusitis, bronchitis and other respiratory tract disorders. However, since these disorders are seldom caused by type b organisms, their incidence will not be affected by Hib vaccines.

The risk of Hib meningitis is at least twice as high for children attending full-time day care as for children cared for at home. The risk is also increased among children with splenic dysfunction (e.g., sickle cell disease, asplenia) or antibody deficiency, and among Inuit children.

Preparations Used for Immunization

All Canadian provinces and territories include Hib conjugate vaccine in their immunization program for children. Hib conjugate vaccines are the second generation of vaccines against Hib disease, having replaced an earlier polysaccharide product. Polysaccharide-protein conjugate antigens have the advantage of producing greater immune response in infants and young children than purified polysaccharide vaccine. The latter stimulates only B-cells, whereas the former activates macrophages, T-helper cells and B-cells, resulting in greatly enhanced antibody responses and establishment of immunologic memory.

As of 1997 three Hib conjugate vaccines are licensed for use in Canada in infants ≥ 2 months of age: HbOC (HibTITER™), PRP-OMP (PedvaxHIB™) and PRP-T (Act-HIB™). A fourth Hib conjugate vaccine, PRP-D (ProHIBIT™), is licensed only for use in children ≥ 18 months of age. However PRP-D is currently not recommended in Canada because it induces antibody responses that are suboptimal compared with other Hib conjugate vaccines.

The Hib conjugate vaccines differ in a number of ways, including the protein carrier, polysaccharide size and types of diluent and preservative. As of 1997, all Canadian provinces and territories use the PRP-T vaccine because it is the only Hib conjugate vaccine currently licensed for use in combination with acellular pertussis vaccine, diphtheria and tetanus toxoids, with or without inactivated polio vaccine.

HbOC, PRP-OMP and PRP-T stimulate good antibody responses after primary immunization in infants starting at 2 to 3 months of age and prime them for an excellent booster response at 15 to 18 months. The booster response can be elicited by any of the conjugate Hib vaccines.

When given as a single dose to previously unimmunized children ≥ 15 months of age, HbOC, PRP-OMP and PRP-T stimulate excellent antibody responses (> 1 µg/mL) in 80% to 100% of children.

The duration of immunity following completion of age-appropriate immunization is unknown and warrants ongoing study. Current data suggest that protection will be long lasting.

Capsular polysaccharide antigen can be detected in the urine of vaccinees for up to 2 weeks after vaccination with conjugate vaccine. This phenomenon could be confused with antigenuria associated with invasive Hib infections.

Hib conjugate vaccine failure, defined as onset of confirmed invasive Hib infection more than 28 days after completion of the primary immunization series, can occur but is rare with the products in current use.

Storage requirements
Hib conjugate vaccines should be stored between 2° and 8°C. Do not freeze. Vaccines that require reconstitution should be used immediately thereafter.

Recommended Usage
Routine immunization with Hib conjugate vaccine is recommended for all infants beginning at 2 months of age. The recommended schedule for PRP-T vaccine is shown in Table 1 along with the schedules for other licensed products. Infants and children starting a primary series of Hib vaccines after 2 months of age should be immunized as soon as possible according to the schedules shown in Table 1. It is preferable when possible to use the same product for all doses in the primary series. However, available data suggest that primary vaccination series consisting of three doses of different Hib conjugate vaccine products result in adequate antibody responses. When use of a different product is unavoidable, for instance, when a child moves from a jurisdiction using different Hib vaccines, the specific vaccine given for each of the primary series injections should be carefully documented.

Haemophilus Vaccine

Protective serum antibody (anti-PRP) concentrations are achieved in 99% of children after completion of the primary PRP-T vaccination series of three doses. However, antibody levels subsequently decline, necessitating a booster dose at 15 to 16 months of age with any of the Hib conjugate vaccines approved for use in infants.

Table 1
Detailed Vaccination Schedule for *Haemophilus* b Conjugate Vaccines

Vaccine	Age at 1st dose (months)	Primary series	Age at booster dose* (months)
PRP-T† (Pasteur Mérieux Connaught)	2-6	3 doses, 2 months apart	15-18
	7-11	2 doses, 2 months apart	15-18
	12-14	1 dose	15-18
	15-59	1 dose	
HbOC‡ (Wyeth Ayerst)	2-6	3 doses, 2 months apart	15-18
	7-11	2 doses, 2 months apart	15-18
	12-14	1 dose	15-18
	15-59	1 dose	
PRP OMP** (Merck-Frosst)	2-6	2 doses, 2 months apart	12
	7-11	2 doses, 2 months apart	15-18
	12-14	1 dose	15-18
	15-59	1 dose	

* The booster dose should be given at least 2 months after the previous dose.
† Supplied as lyophilized powder that can be reconstituted with any of the following Pasteur Mérieux Connaught products: the supplied diluent, DPT adsorbed, DPT polio adsorbed or Quadracel™
‡ Supplied as a solution (HibTITER™) for injection in a separate limb from other vaccines or as a premixed liquid formulation in combination with Wyeth Ayerst DPT adsorbed (TETRAMUNE™)
** Supplied as lyophilized powder that must be reconstituted only with the supplied Merck Frosst diluent

Previously unimmunized children 15 to 59 months of age should be given a single dose of PRP-T, HbOC or PRP-OMP.

Children in whom invasive Hib disease develops before 24 months of age should still receive vaccine as recommended, since natural disease may not induce protection.

Infections due to encapsulated bacteria, including *Haemophilus influenzae*, occur more commonly in persons with disorders of the humoral immune system, both primary and secondary (the latter consisting of disorders of antibody production or function, including lymphoreticular or hematopoietic malignancies, antibody dyscrasias, protein wasting syndromes, anatomic or functional asplenia, bone marrow transplantation and HIV infection). For children who have one of these conditions and who have already received the primary Hib vaccination series plus booster, it is not known whether additional doses of Hib vaccine are beneficial. For previously unimmunized children older than 5 years, or adults, who have underlying conditions that predispose to infection with encapsulated bacteria, the efficacy of Hib vaccination is unknown. Despite limited efficacy data, Hib vaccination is commonly given to those with anatomic or functional asplenia, and may be considered in other immunocompromised persons at increased risk for invasive Hib infection. Consultation with an infectious disease expert may be helpful in these cases.

Hib conjugate vaccines that are supplied as a lyophilized powder should be reconstituted only with products supplied by the same manufacturer, as recommended in product monographs. PRP-T and HbOC may be combined with other vaccines produced by their respective manufacturers. Combined vaccine products allow the administration of multiple antigens with the use of a single needle and have safety profiles similar to those of separately administered vaccines.

Conjugate vaccines should be administered intramuscularly. Any of the four Hib conjugate vaccines may be given simultaneously with oral polio, measles, mumps, rubella, hepatitis B, pneumococcal and meningococcal vaccines but at a different site. There are no data on administration of Hib conjugate vaccines at the same time as influenza vaccine.

The protein carriers in Hib conjugate vaccines should not be considered as immunizing agents against diphtheria, tetanus or meningococcal disease.

Rifampin or other appropriate chemoprophylaxis is not required for household contacts of index cases of invasive Hib infection when the contacts are completely immunized against Hib. Complete immunization is defined as receipt of the primary Hib vaccination series and booster dose as presented in Table 1. When contacts who are less than 48 months of age are not completely immunized, consultation with the local public health unit is advised.

Adverse Reactions

Temperature of more than 38.3° C and localized redness and swelling have been reported in a minority of infants given Hib conjugate vaccine either alone or in combination with other vaccines. No severe adverse reactions have been noted in clinical trials, although a few temporally associated allergic reactions have been reported in older children receiving the vaccine as part of their routine vaccination program.

Contraindications

Vaccination is contraindicated in people who are allergic to any component of the vaccine.

SELECTED REFERENCES

Aderson EL, Decker MD, Englund JA et al. *Interchangeability of conjugated* **Haemophilus influenzae** *type b vaccines in infants.* JAMA 1995;273:849-53.

Committee on Infectious Diseases. **Haemophilus influenzae** *infections.* In: *Report of the Committee of Infectious Diseases (Red Book)*, 24th ed. Elk Grove Village, IL: American Academy of Pediatrics, 1997:220-31.

Eskola J. *Analysis of* **Haemophilus influenzae** *type b conjugate and diphtheria-tetanus-pertussis combination vaccines.* J Infect Dis 1996;174:S302-5.

Friede A, O'Carroll PW, Nicola RM et al, editors. Centers for Disease Control and Prevention. *CDC prevention guidelines. A guide to action.* Baltimore: William and Wilkins, 1997:394-492.

Immunization Monitoring Program, Active (IMPACT) of the Canadian Paediatric Society and the Laboratory Centre for Disease Control. *Recent trends in pediatric* **Haemophilus influenzae** *type b infections in Canada.* Can Med Assoc J 1996;154:1041-47.

LCDC. *Canadian national report on immunization, 1996.* CCDR 1997;23S4:13-4.

LCDC. *Supplementary statement on newly licensed* **Haemophilus influenzae** *type b (HIB) conjugate vaccines in combination with other vaccines recommended for infants (NACI).* CCDR 1994;20:157-60.

Scheifele D, Gold R, Marchessault V et al. *Failures after immunization with* **Haemophilus influenzae** *type b vaccines 1991-1995.* CCDR 1996;2217-23.

Scheifele D, Law B, Mitchell L, Ochnio J. *Study of booster doses of two* **Haemophilus influenzae** *type b conjugate vaccines including their interchangeability.* Vaccine 1996;14:1399-1406.

HEPATITIS A VACCINE

Hepatitis A, previously known as infectious or short-incubation hepatitis, results from infection of the liver by hepatitis A virus (HAV), an RNA virus of a single serotype. Infection usually causes overt illness in adults and school-age children but is often asymptomatic in younger children. Humans are the principal reservoir for the virus. Typical symptoms of illness include anoxeria, nausea, fatigue, fever and jaundice. Recovery often takes 4 to 6 weeks. About 25% of reported adult cases require hospitalization. Fulminant disease with liver necrosis is rare but can be fatal. The estimated mortality rate due to hepatitis A in hospitalized adults is 0.14%. Individuals with pre-existing chronic liver disease are at increased risk of serious complications from hepatitis A infection.

Persistent infection does not occur. Spread of hepatitis A occurs by the fecal-oral route, through direct contact with infected persons or indirectly through ingestion of contaminated water or foods, especially uncooked shellfish. The incubation period ranges from 15 to 50 days with an average of 20 to 30 days. Maximum infectivity occurs during the latter part of the incubation period prior to the onset of jaundice. Lifelong immunity usually follows infection.

Risk factors for infection in Canada include the following:

■ residence in certain communities in rural or remote areas lacking adequate sanitation

■ residence in certain institutions, such as correctional facilities and those for developmentally challenged persons

■ oral or intravenous illicit drug use

■ male homosexual behaviours involving anal contact

■ travel to or residence in countries with inadequate sanitation

Cases in returned travellers and contacts of travellers account for a large proportion of reported cases in some areas. The risk for susceptible travellers to developing countries has been estimated at 3 to 5 per 1,000 per month, increasing in persons eating or drinking under poor hygienic conditions. Between 1990 and 1995, the annual number of cases of HAV infection reported to the National Notifiable Disease Registry System has varied from 1,712 to 3,020 (mean 2,217) with corresponding rates from 5.9 to 11.2 (mean 7.9) per 100,000. However, given underreporting and asymptomatic infection, the actual number of cases is considerably higher. In 1995 the reported rate was 1.5 times higher in males than females. Age-specific rates were highest for those <15 years of age and lowest for those > 59 years of age; 32% of all cases were

■ Hepatitis A Vaccine

< 15 years, an age group in which the disease is often asymptomatic (Figure 1). Although representative data are not available for the general Canadian population, studies indicate that immunity to HAV infection is evident in about 3% of Canadian-born preadolescents and in over 60% of those > 59 years of age. The difference in experience between these ages reflects progressive diminution of infection risk with improving social conditions. Overall, the most commonly identified risk factor for HAV infection is household or sexual exposure to a recent case. In many infected persons no specific risk factor can be identified. In Canada, unlike the U.S., there is little evidence of risk of HAV infection in children or staff associated with child day-care facilities in the absence of community outbreaks.

Figure 1: Reported Hepatitis A Cases and Rates by Age Group, Canada, 1995 (National Notifiable Disease Registry System)

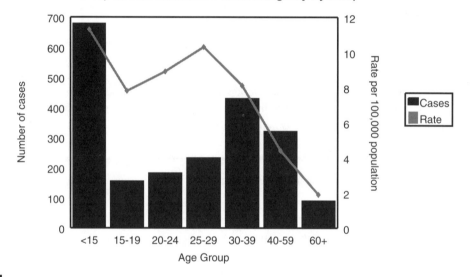

Preparations Used for Immunization

Currently two inactivated hepatitis A vaccines are licensed in Canada along with a combined hepatitis A and hepatitis B vaccine (Table 1). Cell-culture-adapted virus is propagated in human fibroblasts, purified from cell lysates, inactivated with formalin and adsorbed to an aluminum hydroxide adjuvant.

If the second dose in the hepatitis A vaccine series is missed it can be given at any time without repeat of the first dose. It is probable that either product could be used for the second dose, if necessary; however, supporting data are lacking.

Table 1
Schedule and Dosages of Hepatitis A Vaccines

Vaccine	Composition	Vaccine series
Havrix 1440 (Smith Kline Beecham)	1440 ELISA units/mL inactivated hepatitis A antigen	2 doses, the second 6-12 months after the first*
Havrix 720 junior (1-18 years)	720 ELISA units/mL inactivated hepatitis A antigen (Both formulations contain 2-phenoxyethanol as preservative and trace amounts of neomycin.)	2 doses, the second 6-12 months after the first
Vaqta (Merck Frosst)	50 U hepatitis A virus antigen per/mL dose	2 doses, the second 6 months after the first
Pediatric formulation	25 U hepatitis A virus antigen per 0.5 mL dose (Both formulations may contain residual formaldehyde and neomycin.)	2 doses, the second 6-18 months after the first
Twinrix (Smith Kline Beecham)	Havrix 720 ELISA units and Engerix B 20 µg of purified hepatitis B surface antigen protein in 1 mL	3 doses at 0, 1 and 6 months
Pediatric formulation	Havrix 360 ELISA units and 10 µg of purified hepatitis B surface antigen protein in 0.5 mL	

* When Havrix 1440 is used for the primary dose, evidence from previous studies has shown that a dose of 720 ELISA units provides an effective booster response in adults.

Epidemiologic studies of hepatitis A outbreaks have shown that no cases occurred 3 weeks or more after vaccination, suggesting that receipt of vaccine prior to exposure is almost invariably protective. In serologic studies 97%-99% of individuals developed protective levels ($\geq$ 10 IU/mL) of serum antibody against HAV 4 weeks after primary immunization with inactivated hepatitis A vaccine. In healthy adults 88% had serum antibody against HAV measurable by enzyme-linked immunosorbent assay (ELISA) 2 weeks after a primary dose of Havrix 1440®. Two weeks after vaccination with Vaqta® 69% of adults tested had anti-HAV levels of $\geq$ 10 IU/mL.

After the second dose of vaccine the duration of protection and thus the need for additional booster doses is unknown, but kinetic models of antibody decline suggest that protective levels of antibody may persist for at least 20 years. The high response rate to vaccination makes routine serologic testing after vaccination unnecessary.

Hepatitis A vaccine should be stored between 2° and 8° C and should not be frozen. Opened vials of Vaqta® should be used promptly since they contain no preservative. Hepatitis A vaccines should be administered intramuscularly.

Recommended Usage
Pre-exposure prophylaxis
Hepatitis A vaccine is recommended for pre-exposure prophylaxis of individuals at increased risk of infection. Potential candidates for the vaccine are

■ travellers to countries where hepatitis A is endemic, especially when travel involves rural or primitive conditions;

■ residents of communities with high endemic rates or recurrent outbreaks of HAV;

■ members of the armed forces, emergency relief workers and others likely to be posted abroad at short notice to areas with high rates of HAV infection;

■ residents and staff of institutions for the developmentally challenged where there is an ongoing problem with HAV transmission;

■ inmates of correctional facilities in which there is an ongoing problem with HAV infection;

■ people with life-style determined risks of infection, including those engaging in oral or intravenous illicit drug use in unsanitary conditions;

■ men who have sex with men;

■ people with chronic liver disease who may not be at increased risk of infection but are at increased risk of fulminant hepatitis A; and

■ others, such as patients with hemophilia A or B receiving plasma-derived replacement clotting factors (the solvent-detergent method used to prepare all the present plasma-derived factor VIII and some factor IX concentrates does not reliably inactivate HAV, a non-enveloped virus); zoo-keepers, veterinarians and researchers who handle non-human primates; and certain workers involved in research on hepatitis A virus or production of hepatitis A vaccine.

Outbreak control
Hepatitis A vaccine may be used as part of a coordinated public health response to hepatitis A outbreaks. The vaccine may be used on a community-wide basis to prevent infection and to halt the spread of infection. There is insufficient evidence to determine the level of protection afforded by the vaccine if given after exposure. Studies suggest that concomitant administration of immune globulin (IG) with hepatitis A vaccine reduces antibody levels; however, this reduction is not thought to be clinically significant.

At present, people in the following circumstances do not need routine vaccination:

- Children and staff of child-care facilities. Although such facilities have often been the focus of outbreaks in the United States, such events have not been frequently reported in Canada. In addition, serologic testing has not indicated an increased risk of infection for workers or children.

- Health care workers are not considered to be at increased risk if standard infection control techniques can be exercised. Data from serosurveys of health care workers have not shown a greater prevalence of HAV infection.

- Sewage workers may be at increased risk of infection during community outbreaks, but the data are insufficient to make a recommendation for routine vaccination.

- Food handlers may be a source of foodborne outbreaks of hepatitis A but are not themselves at increased risk of infection. It has not been determined to what extent vaccination of such workers would be practical or effective in reducing foodborne outbreaks.

Adverse Reactions and Contraindications

Side effects reported in vaccine recipients are generally mild and transient, and limited to soreness and redness at the injection site. Local side effects in children appear to be less frequent than in adults. No significant difference in symptoms is evident between initial and subsequent doses or in the presence of pre-existing immunity. Rare instances of anaphylaxis have been reported.

The safety of HAV vaccine given during pregnancy has not been established. Since the vaccine is prepared from inactivated virus the risk to the developing fetus is likely to be negligible; however, it should not be given to pregnant women unless there is a definite risk of infection.

Immune Globulin

Immune globulin will provide protection against hepatitis A when administered intramuscularly before exposure or during the incubation period. Its relative effectiveness depends upon both the timing of administration and the dose given. Hepatitis A vaccine is the preferable method of pre-exposure prophylaxis against hepatitis A; however, IG may be indicated for infants < 1 year and individuals for whom the vaccine is contraindicated.

The recommended doses of IG vary according to the duration of required protection:[1]
< 3 months: 0.02 mL/kg
3-5 months: 0.06 mL/kg
> 5 months: 0.06 mL/kg prior to exposure and then every 5 months if exposure continues.

---

[1]   varies with manufacturer – consult package insert

For post-exposure prophylaxis, IG should be given as soon as possible after known exposure. It is of greatest value when given early in the incubation period and of little or no value when given more than 2 weeks after exposure. Individuals who have received hepatitis A vaccine before exposure according to the recommended schedule do not need IG prophylaxis. The recommended dose is 0.02 mL/kg and should be offered to the following:

- all household contacts of cases of acute hepatitis A;

- children and employees of day-care centres as indicated below

    day-care centres that accept diapered children
    IG should be given to all children and employees of the centre if one case occurs in an attendee or staff member, or if cases occur in at least two families of attendees. Family members of children < 4 years of age attending such a day-care centre should also be considered for prophylaxis if the outbreak is recognized more than 3 weeks after onset or if cases have occurred in three or more families of attendees.

    day-care facilities not for diapered children
    IG need be administered only to close contacts of the index case.

- residents and staff of institutions in which an outbreak is occurring.

Routine administration of IG is not recommended for health care workers in contact with an infected patient or for workers in contact with a case in offices or factories. Use in schools for pupils or teachers in contact with a case is not indicated unless there is evidence of ongoing transmission in the school or classroom. In common-source outbreaks and community wide outbreaks of hepatitis A in open populations, recognition of the source usually occurs too late to allow administration of IG to be of value.

Immunization of Travellers

Vaccination against hepatitis A is recommended for travellers to and people planning to live in developing countries, especially in rural areas or where the hygienic quality of the food and water supply is likely to be poor, and in areas where hepatitis A is endemic. Active immunization with hepatitis A vaccine is the first choice for protection against hepatitis A for travellers. Given the good serologic response to vaccine after the primary dose, simultaneous administration of IG is not indicated even if the vaccine is given immediately before departure. IG may be used for infants < 1 year and individuals for whom the vaccine is contraindicated.

SELECTED REFERENCES

Allard R, Durand L, Guy M, Deshaies D, Robert J. *Hepatitis A in downtown Montreal, Quebec, 1990-1992.* CCDR 1995;21:71-6.

CDC. *Prevention of hepatitis A through active or passive immunization: recommendations of the Advisory Committee on Immunization Practices.* MMWR 1996;45:RR-15.

De Serres G, Laliberte D. *Hepatitis A among workers from a waste water treatment plant during a small community outbreak.* Occup Environ Med 1997;54:60-2.

Kocuipchyk MF, Lightfoot PJ, Stout I, Devine RD. *Seroprevalence of hepatitis A antibodies in travellers at the Edmonton Traveller's Health Clinic Alberta.* CCDR 1995;21:65-71.

LCDC. *National notifiable diseases annual summary 1995.* CCDR 1997;23S9:1-104.

Lemon SM, Thomas DL. *Vaccines to prevent viral hepatitis.* N Engl J Med 1997;336:196-204.

National Advisory Committee on Immunization. *Statement on the prevention of hepatitis A infections.* CCDR 1994;20:133-36, 139-43.

National Advisory Committee on Immunization. *Supplementary statement on hepatitis A prevention.* CCDR 1996;22:1-3.

National Advisory Committee on Immunization. *Supplementary statement on hepatitis prevention.* CCDR 1997;23(ACS-4):1-6.

Ochnio JJ, Scheifele DW, Ho M. *Hepatitis A virus infections in urban children – are preventive opportunities being missed?* J Infect Dis 1997;176:1610-13.

Payment P. *Antibody levels to selected enteric viruses in a French-Canadian population in the province of Quebec (Canada).* Immunol Infect Dis 1991;1:317-22.

Vento S, Garofano T, Renzini C et al. *Fulminant hepatitis associated with hepatitis A virus superinfection in patients with chronic hepatitis C.* N Engl J Med 1998;388:286-90.

HEPATITIS B VACCINE

Hepatitis B virus (HBV) is one of several viruses that cause hepatitis. HBV is a double stranded DNA virus with three major antigens known as hepatitis B surface antigen (HBsAg), hepatitis B e antigen (HBeAg) and hepatitis B core antigen (HBcAg). The presence of HBsAg can be detected in serum 30 to 60 days after exposure and persists until the infection resolves. The incubation period for hepatitis B is 45 to 160 days (average 120 days). Antibody to hepatitis B surface antigen (anti-HBs) appears in serum after the infection has resolved and confers long-term immunity. In a proportion of cases, which varies inversely with age, infection persists and this protective antibody is not produced. HBcAg never appears in serum. Anti-HBc develops in all HBV infections, is not protective and persists indefinitely. Anti-HBc IgM is a marker of recent HBV infection. HBeAg in serum is associated with viral replication and high levels of infectiousness. Anti-HBe indicates loss of replicating virus and lower infectiousness. Any serum containing HBsAg, however, is considered infectious.

HBV infection is usually associated with exposure to blood or infectious bodily fluids. Common means of transmission include heterosexual and homosexual contact, injection drug use, and perinatal transmission (mother to infant). The risk of transfusion-related hepatitis B is extremely low because of routine HBsAg screening of donated blood and rejection of donors at risk of infection. Infections also occur in settings of close personal contact through unrecognized contact with infective fluids. In about 35% of cases, no risk factors can be identified.

Initial infection with HBV may be asymptomatic in up to 50% of cases, or symptomatic. Acute illness may last up to 3 months and has a case-fatality rate of 1% to 2%. An individual with either acute symptomatic or asymptomatic HBV infection may become a chronic carrier. A chronic carrier is an individual from whom serum samples taken 6 months apart are HBsAg positive or a single serum sample is HBsAg positive and anti-HBc IgM negative. The risk of becoming a chronic carrier varies inversely with the age at which infection occurs (infants 90% to 95% risk; children < 5 years 25% to 50%; adults 6% to 10%). The risk of becoming a chronic carrier is also greater in immunocompromised patients. Chronic carriers often do not have overt disease, but over time are at increased risk for hepatic cirrhosis and hepatocellular carcinoma. Chronic carriers are likely the major source of infection, and all carriers should be considered infectious.

Although there are no national data on the prevalence of chronic HBV infection for the whole Canadian population, Canada is considered an area of low endemicity. It is estimated that less than 5% of residents have markers of past infection and less than 0.5% are HBsAg carriers. There are, however, specific segments of the population that have increased risk for HBV infection and consequently higher prevalence of infection. These segments include populations with the following risk factors:

- Lifestyle risk factors, including male homosexuality and injection drug use

- Geographic risk factors, including infection acquired in economically disadvantaged parts of the world, where the prevalence of HBV is higher than in Canada, and in some Native populations

- Occupational risk factors, such as health care workers exposed frequently to blood. In some of these populations, such as health care workers, the risk of infection has been reduced with the use of HBV vaccine.

Although the rate of HBV infection reported to the National Notifiable Diseases Registry System (NNDRS) increased more than 100% from 1980 to 1990, the rates of new HBV infection reached a plateau in the 1990s (Figure 1). The interpretation of these data is clouded by the fact that there has been inconsistency in reporting acute versus chronic infections, and that the data are driven by the large number of cases from British Columbia, which reported 44% of all cases in Canada from 1990 to 1995. When the data are restricted to acute HBV infection, there is a significant downward trend in incidence between 1992 and 1995 for each age group between 15 and 59 years of age (Figure 2). The age-specific rates are low for those < 15 years of age, rising rapidly to a peak for those 25 to 29 years, and then declining to low rates for those over 59 years of age. These data imply that sexual activity and injection drug use continue to play important roles in HBV transmission in Canada.

Figure 1: Annual Crude Rates of Hepatitis B in Canada, 1992-1995, As Reported by NNDRS* and for "Acute Hepatitis B"

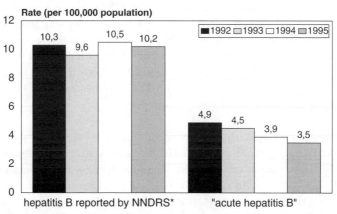

*NNDRS=National Notifiable Diseases Registry System

Figure 2: Annual Rates for "Acute Hepatitis B" in Canada, 1992-1995, by Age Group

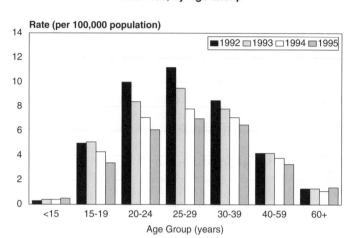

Rate (per 100,000 population)

Age Group (years)

■1992 ☐1993 ☐1994 ■1995

<15 15-19 20-24 25-29 30-39 40-59 60+

Preparations Used for Immunization

Hepatitis B vaccines contain purified recombinant HBsAg and induce anti-HBs production, which confers immunity to hepatitis B. Hepatitis B vaccines are licensed in Canada for pre-exposure and post-exposure prophylaxis. Antigenic subtypes of HBV exist, but immunization confers immunity to all subtypes because of the presence of a common antigen.

Two recombinant DNA hepatitis B vaccines are licensed in Canada, one prepared by Merck Sharp and Dohme (Recombivax HB®) and the other by SmithKline Beecham (Engerix-B®). Both vaccines are produced from a genetically engineered yeast strain. Recombivax HB contains 10 µg/mL and Engerix-B® 20 µg/mL of purified hepatitis B surface antigen. A preparation of Recombivax® HB containing 40 µg/mL is available for use in patients who receive hemodialysis. The vaccines are adsorbed onto aluminum hydroxide with thimerosal as preservative. Trace amounts of yeast antigens are present in the vaccines, but no increase in yeast antibody titres has been observed following administration of either vaccine. The vaccines are well tolerated, and reactions are usually mild.

Twinrix® (SmithKline Beecham) is a bivalent vaccine containing 20 µg of purified hepatitis B surface antigen protein and 720 ELISA units of inactivated hepatitis A viral antigen (HM 175 strain) in one millilitre. The manufacturer recommends its use in persons at risk of both hepatitis A and B, to be given at 0, 1 and 6 months. All recipients show protective antibody against hepatitis A and almost all against hepatitis B 1 month after the third dose.

The standard preparation of plasma-derived hepatitis B vaccine has not been available in Canada since August of 1990, and the preparation used for dialysis patients has not been available since February 1991.

Schedule and Dosages

The recommended schedule for hepatitis B vaccine is three doses given at 0, 1 and 6 months. There is evidence that the closer the last dose is given to 12 months after the first, the greater and longer lasting the antibody response will be. An alternative four-dose schedule for Engerix-B® at 0, 1, 2 and 12 months may result in earlier protection. There is no benefit in giving the last dose later than 12 months after the first, except possibly in the case of infants. A variety of schedules used in Canada and throughout the world are valid for infants and others, and may be used to administer vaccine to infants at regular well-baby visits.

Interruption of the immunization schedule does not require that any dose be repeated, as long as the minimum intervals between doses are respected. If any dose has not been given according to an approved schedule, it should be given at the first opportunity. If years have elapsed between dose one and dose two, it may be prudent to assess antibody response when the series is complete, especially if the patient is at significant risk of infection.

The dose of vaccine administered varies with age, the product used and some medical conditions (see Table 1). Doses of 40 µg are recommended for adult hemodialysis patients. For children receiving hemodialysis, the common practice is to double the dose for the child's age and assess the antibody response when the series is complete. Infants weighing < 2000 g born to infected mothers should have an individualized schedule that includes at least four doses of vaccine, HBIG, and assessment of antibody response after the series has been completed.

Vaccines produced by different manufacturers can be used interchangeably despite different doses and schedules. The dose used should be that recommended by the manufacturer.

Hepatitis B immune globulin (HBIG) (see page 182) is prepared from pooled human plasma from selected donors with a high level of anti-HBs who are seronegative for bloodborne infections. HBIG provides immediate and effective short-term passive immunity. HBIG administered concurrently with vaccine, but at a different site, does not interfere with the antibody response.

Table 1

Recommended Doses of Currently Licensed Hepatitis B Vaccines

Recipients	Recombivax HB®		Engerix-B®	
	µg	mL	µg	mL
Infants of HBV-carrier mothers	5.0	0.5	10	0.5
Infants of HBV-negative mothers and children ≤ 10 years	2.5	0.25	10	0.5
Children 11 to 19 years	5.0	0.5	10	0.5
Adults	10	1.0	20	1.0
Hemodialysis and immuno-compromised patients	40	1.0*	40	2.0

* When special formulation is used.

Route of Vaccine Administration

All hepatitis B vaccines should be injected into the deltoid muscle of children and adults, and into the anterolateral thigh muscle of infants. Gluteal administration should not be used because of poor immune response, possibly the result of inadvertent deposition into fatty tissue. Use of vaccine that has been frozen or inadequately mixed has also led to poor antibody responses.

Immune responses following intradermal injection have been variable, and this route of vaccine administration is not recommended.

Hepatitis B vaccine may be administered simultaneously with other vaccines at different sites. A separate needle and syringe should be used for each vaccine.

Response Rate to Immunization

Use of the recommended schedule and routes of immunization results in seroconversion rates of 90% to 95% in immunocompetent individuals. The antibody response rate is lower in immunocompromised patients, such as those infected with HIV (50% to 70%), patients with renal failure (60% to 70%), diabetes mellitus (70%

to 80%) and chronic liver disease (60% to 70%). Vaccination of smokers and people with alcoholism produces lower antibody titres than in others.

Antibody response is also age related. Children between age 2 and 19 years have the highest response rate (99%), and children < 2 years of age have a 95% response rate. The response rate decreases in adults: 20 to 29 years 95%, 30 to 39 years 90%, 40 to 49 years 86%, 50 to 59 years 71% and > 60 years 50% to 70%.

Recommended Usage

Hepatitis B prevention should include programs for universal immunization of children, pre-exposure vaccination of high-risk groups, universal HBsAg screening of all pregnant women and post-exposure intervention for those exposed to disease, particularly infants born to HBV-infected mothers.

1. Universal immunization

NACI recommends that a universal immunization program during childhood be implemented to control HBV infection. The Canadian Hepatitis B Working Group has recommended that a pre-adolescent strategy be used, because it is the most cost-effective option and because very few hepatitis B infections occur in young children. Should effective combination vaccines that include hepatitis B in addition to the other childhood vaccines become available in Canada for infants, NACI would support their use.

If childhood immunization against HBV is given in infancy, the level and duration of protection may be better if the last dose is given after the first birthday. Because of the possibility of false positive laboratory results, an unimmunized child who is positive for either anti-HBs or anti-HBc should still receive hepatitis B vaccine.

It is further recommended that any person who wants protection against HBV should be encouraged to receive hepatitis B vaccine.

2. Health care and emergency service workers and other occupational exposure

Immunization with hepatitis B vaccine is recommended for those persons who are at increased risk of occupational infection, namely, those exposed frequently to blood, blood products and bodily fluids that may contain the virus. This group includes all health care workers and others who will be or may be exposed to blood or are at risk of injury by blood-contaminated instruments. For these workers, a series of injections of hepatitis B vaccine should be initiated at the first opportunity. Students in these occupations should complete their vaccine series before possible occupational exposure to blood or sharps injuries. Emergency service workers, such as police and firefighters, may also be at higher risk of exposure, although there are currently no data to quantify their risk. Workers who have no contact with blood or blood products are at no greater risk than the general population.

3. Others at increased risk

a. Residents and staff of institutions for the developmentally disabled.

b. Homosexual and bisexual males.

c. Heterosexual males or females with multiple sexual partners or with a recent history of a sexually transmitted disease.

d. Injection drug users.

e. Hemophiliacs and others receiving repeated infusions of blood or blood products.

f. Hemodialysis patients. Adults require 40 µg of vaccine antigen per dose. A specific formulation for dialysis is available (Recombivax 40 µg per mL) to be given at 0, 1 and 6 months. When the required dosage is achieved using two adult vials of Engerix B (20 µg per mL each), a series of four immunizations at 0, 1, 2 and 6 months is recommended by the manufacturer.

g. Inmates of long-term correctional facilities.

h. Household and sexual contacts of acute HBV cases and HBV carriers; people who do not live in the same household, apart from sexual contacts, need not be considered for vaccination.

i. Populations or communities in which HBV is highly endemic.

j. Children < 7 years of age whose families have immigrated to Canada from areas where there is a high prevalence of hepatitis B, and who are exposed to HBV carriers through their extended families.

k. Travellers to hepatitis B endemic areas.

l. Children in child care settings in which there is an HBV-infected child. These children should receive serious consideration for immunization against HBV.

4. Post-exposure prophylaxis

a. Infants: In view of the importance of preventing hepatitis B infection in infants, all pregnant women should be routinely tested for HBsAg. All infants born to infected mothers should be given an intramuscular dose of 0.5 mL HBIG immediately after birth and a course of three doses of hepatitis B vaccine. The initial dose should be given as soon as possible but no later than 7 days after birth (see Table 1). It is important that HBIG also be given as soon as possible but within the first few hours of birth since efficacy decreases sharply after 48 hours. Vaccine and HBIG may be given at the same time but at different sites. The second and third dose of the vaccine series should be given 1 and 6 months after the first. For neonates < 2000 g, an additional dose of vaccine 2 months after the third dose is recommended. Accountability mechanisms should be in place to ensure that every infant born to an infected mother receives HBIG, a full course of vaccine and testing for serologic response to the vaccine.

If testing has not been done during pregnancy, it should be done on an urgent basis at the time of delivery. If maternal HBV status is not available within 12 hours after delivery, consideration should be given to administering HBIG while the results are pending, *taking into account the mother's risk factors.* If the mother is shown to have HBV infection, a series of vaccine doses should also be given. Should the mother's infection be recognized during lactation, the infant's HBV status should be assessed urgently and the infant started immediately on full immunoprophylaxis, which should be completed if the infant is found not to be already infected or immune.

When a mother is infected with HBV, testing of the infant for HBsAg and anti-HBs is recommended 1 month after completion of vaccination to monitor the success of this prophylaxis. If HBsAg is found, the child is likely to become a chronic carrier. If the infant is negative for both HBsAg and anti-HBs (i.e., a non-responder), a fourth dose should be given with repeated serologic testing for antibody response, or the course of vaccine should be repeated.

b. Percutaneous (needlestick) or mucosal exposure: Table 2 outlines the management of vaccinated or unvaccinated individuals after potential exposure to hepatitis B, including injury by needles found on the street. The management of potential percutaneous or mucosal exposure to HBV should be based on the vaccination and antibody status of the injured person and the infectious status, if known, of the source. It is critical to ascertain whether the exposed individual has received a full and properly administered course of hepatitis B vaccine and to determine the post-vaccination anti-HBs antibody level. Therefore, all health care workers and health care students should have their antibody status documented and recorded after immunization. A protective level of antibody is considered to be 10 international units per litre (IU/L) of anti-HBs. Levels above this achieved after immunization correlate with long-term protection even if antibody levels later fall below 10 IU/L.

Testing of the source should be conducted according to the Health Canada 1997 guidelines *An integrated protocol to manage health care workers exposed to bloodborne pathogens.* Informed consent should be obtained and confidentiality respected. If the assessments of the injured person and the source are not available within 48 hours, management of the injured person should assume possible exposure.

Table 2
Post-Exposure Immunoprophylaxis for Hepatitis B

This table recommends action for possible exposure to hepatitis B according to the vaccination and antibody status of the exposed person. The source may be known to be infected or in a risk group for infection, or infectious status may not be known, either because the source has not been identified or has not been tested. The recommendations assume the real possibility of exposure in ways in which HBV is known to be transmitted.

Vaccination and antibody status of the exposed person:

a. **immunized with documented protective anti-HBs at any time or documented as immune because of previous natural infection**
   – no action required

b. **no anti-HBs response to two previous courses of vaccine**
   – administer HBIG
   – assess for HBV infection at least 2 months after the exposure

c. **two or more doses of vaccine; anti-HBs status not known**
   i) health care workers or others known or highly likely to have been exposed to HBV
   – test for anti-HBs and simultaneously administer one dose of vaccine*
   – if the first test is negative, retest 4 weeks after this dose, and if still negative assess for HBV infection at least 2 months after the exposure
   – give the final dose of a three-dose series at the time it is normally due if infection has not occurred and anti-HBs is still lacking
   ii) all others
   – test for anti-HBs as soon as possible
   – if negative, administer one dose of vaccine*
   – retest 4 weeks after this dose, and if still negative assess for HBV infection at least 2 months after the exposure
   – give the final dose at the time it is normally due if infection has not occurred

d. **0 or 1 dose of vaccine or non-responder to one course of vaccine**
   – administer HBIG and an accelerated course of vaccine at 0, 1, 2 and 6 to 12 months
   – assess for HBV infection at least 2 months after the exposure

* HBIG will be of value only in the unlikely situation that the source is infected and the worker has no protection despite immunization. It should be given if there is compelling reason to do so.

Notes:

1. If test results are available on the source patient within 48 hours and show that the source is not infected, the use of HBIG may be precluded in b and d above.
2. If the source is known not to be infected or known to be at negligible risk for HBV, the only required action is to ensure that the workers receive the usual pre-exposure course of vaccine and antibody testing if these actions have not already been completed.
3. LCDC recommends baseline testing of the health care worker for HBsAg and anti-HBs; testing for anti-HBc is recommended if the injured HCW is susceptible, a non-responder, or has an unknown anti-HBs status at the time of injury; if tests are negative, retesting after 6 months is recommended.
4. This advice differs from the 1997 statement published in the CCDR supplement in the following ways: This table is based primarily on the status of the injured health care worker and not the source. In the CCDR supplement HBIG is recommended for health care workers who have unknown anti-HBs status; a second dose 1 month after the first is recommended if the health care worker is a known non-responder.

c. Sexual and household contacts of hepatitis B: All sexual and household contacts of acute cases and chronic carriers should be vaccinated.

Sexual partners of an acute case or carrier of hepatitis B should complete a hepatitis B vaccine series. If prophylaxis can be started within 14 days of the last sexual contact with the HBV-infected person, a single dose of HBIG (0.06 mL/kg) should also be given. Sexual assault victims should be managed in the same manner if the HBsAg status of the assailant cannot be ascertained.

All sexual partners of people with HBV infection should be counselled that protection from infection cannot be assured until the course of vaccine has been completed and anti-HBs demonstrated. There should be counselling on the use of condoms and their ability to reduce but not eliminate the risk of transmission.

HBIG is not indicated for non-sexual household contacts of an acute HBV case; exceptions are infants < 12 months of age whose mother or primary care giver is acutely or chronically infected and persons with identifiable exposure to the blood of someone with active HBV, as may occur if toothbrushes or razors are shared.

Booster Doses of Vaccine

Routine booster vaccinations in immunocompetent persons are not recommended since protection has been shown to last for at least 15 years. Studies of long-term protective efficacy, however, will determine whether booster doses of vaccine are ever needed. It is important to recognize that absence of detectable anti-HBs in a person who has been previously demonstrated to have anti-HBs does not mean lack of protection, because immune memory persists. Booster doses in this situation are not indicated.

Immunocompromised persons often respond suboptimally to the vaccine. Subsequent HBV exposures in these individuals can result in disease or the carrier state. Therefore, boosters may be necessary in this population. The optimal timing of booster doses for immunocompromised individuals who are at continued risk of HBV exposure is not known and should be based on the severity of the compromised state and annual monitoring for the presence of anti-HBs.

Serologic Testing for Hepatitis B Antigen and Antibody

Pregnancy: All pregnant women should be routinely tested for HBsAg at the first prenatal visit. If testing has not been done during pregnancy, it should be done at the time of delivery. Repeat testing prior to delivery may be considered in women with continuing high-risk behaviour. Infants born to HBsAg positive mothers should receive post-exposure prophylaxis.

A pregnant woman who has no markers of acute or chronic HBV infection but who is at high risk of acquiring HBV should be offered HBV vaccination.

Adopted children at high risk: Children adopted from countries, geographic regions or family situations in which there is a high prevalence of HBV infection should be screened for HBsAg. If the results are positive, the household contacts should be immunized, preferably before the adoption.

Pre-vaccination serologic screening for antibody: Routine pre-vaccination serologic testing for hepatitis B, including HBsAg, anti-HBs or anti-HBc, is recommended for persons at high risk of having been infected before immunization. This testing will identify those already infected or immune, for whom vaccine will confer no benefit. Testing will also assist in the medical management and contact follow-up of those individuals found to be infected already, and prevent the mistaken belief that no risk is posed to others. The cost of such testing may or may not be less than the cost of immunization, depending on the HBV prevalence in the high-risk population. Routine serologic screening before vaccination, however, is not practical for universal immunization programs.

Post-vaccination serologic tests: The seroconversion rate after hepatitis B vaccination in healthy people is usually 90% or more, and in children 98% or more. Thus, post-immunization testing for universal programs is not necessary.

Post-immunization testing is recommended, however, if it is important to ensure protection against a continual known or repeated potential exposure to hepatitis B. This would be the case for infants born to infected mothers, sexual partners of chronic carriers, and those who have been immunized because of occupational exposure.

In particular, post-vaccination testing for anti-HBs should be conducted on all health care workers and students in health care disciplines to establish antibody response and the need for reimmunization should the first course of vaccine fail to provide protection. If antibody levels are protective, testing need not be repeated. Results should be recorded in the individual's medical file and provided to the tested person. Determination of antibody response after *reimmunization* will identify those who do not respond to two courses of vaccine and who will need passive immunization after potential exposure to hepatitis B.

In addition, sexual assault victims and those who are immunocompromised should also be tested after the vaccine course is completed. If protective antibody is not present, the vaccine course should be repeated, and if protective antibody is still not present, the individual should receive counselling on alternative risk reduction measures.

Post-vaccination testing, when indicated, should be performed as soon as practical after 1 month but no longer than 6 months after completion of the vaccine series. If post-vaccination testing in a health care worker has not been done in this period, it should be conducted as part of the routine follow up when a potential exposure occurs.

Revaccination of Non-Responders

An additional three dose series will produce a protective antibody response in 50% to 70% of those who fail to show a response after the first series. Individuals who fail to respond to the second three-dose vaccination series are unlikely to benefit from further immunization.

Adverse Reactions and Contraindications

Hepatitis B vaccines are safe to administer to adults and children. Reported side effects are usually mild, transient and generally limited to soreness at the injection site and temperature greater than 37.7° C. Pain occurs no more frequently, however, than with placebo.

As with all vaccines, anaphylaxis is very rare but can occur. The only true contraindication to hepatitis B vaccine is a previous anaphylactic reaction to any component of the vaccine.

Cases of rheumatoid arthritis and demyelinating diseases of the central nervous system have been reported rarely, but a causative link to hepatitis B vaccine has not been identified.

Pregnancy should not be considered a contraindication to use of vaccine for persons in whom immunization is recommended, since acute hepatitis B in a pregnant woman may result in severe disease for the mother and chronic infection of the infant. Although data are not available on the safety of these vaccines for the fetus, the risk is expected to be negligible since the vaccines consist of non-infectious subunits.

Adverse reactions have not been observed when hepatitis B vaccines have been given to persons who are immune to hepatitis B or who are hepatitis B carriers.

SELECTED REFERENCES

Alter MJ, Hadler SC, Margolis HS et al. *The changing epidemiology of hepatitis B in the United States: need for alternative vaccination strategies.* JAMA 1990;263:1218-22.

Bloom BS, Hillman AL, Fendrick AM, Schwartz JS. *A reappraisal of hepatitis B virus vaccination strategies using cost-effectiveness analysis.* Ann Intern Med 1993;118:298-306.

Duval B, Boulianne G, De Serres G. *Should children with isolated anti-HBs or anti-HBc be immunized against hepatitis B virus?* JAMA 1997;287:1064.

Hadler SC, Margolis HS. *Hepatitis B immunisation: vaccine types, efficacy, and indications for immunisation.* In: Remington JS, Swartz MN, eds. *Current clinical topics in infectious diseases.* Cambridge: Blackwell Scientific Publications, 1992:282-308.

LCDC. *An integrated protocol to manage health care workers exposed to bloodborne pathogens.* CCDR 1997;23S2:1-14.

Infectious Disease & Immunization Committee, Canadian Paediatric Society. *Hepatitis B in Canada: the case for universal vaccination.* Can Med Assoc J 1992;146:25-8.

Krahn MD, Detsky AS. *Universal hepatitis B vaccination: the economics of prevention.* Can Med Assoc J 1992;146:19-21.

Salisbury D, Begg, N. *Immunization against infectious disease.* HMSO, 1996.

Tepper M. *Acute hepatitis B incidence in Canada.* CCDR 1997;23:52-5.

INFLUENZA VACCINE

NACI produces a "Statement on Influenza Vaccination" each year that contains specific information on the vaccine to be used in the forthcoming season. It is published in the Canada Communicable Disease Report, and it can also be accessed through a FAXlink service (613-941-3900) or using the Health Canada Website (http://www.hc-sc.gc.ca).

Influenza is caused by influenza A and B viruses and occurs in Canada every year, generally during late fall and the winter months. Influenza A viruses, which periodically undergo antigenic changes, are the most common cause of epidemic influenza. Outbreaks of influenza B are generally more localized and in any 1 year may be restricted to one region of the country. An association between influenza outbreaks, especially those caused by type B virus, and cases of the rare but serious Reye syndrome has been noted.

The annual incidence of influenza varies widely, and it is difficult to predict the impact of a particular virus strain on disease during an inter-pandemic period. Persons at greatest risk of serious disease and death are those with chronic medical conditions (especially cardiopulmonary diseases) and the elderly. Although many other respiratory viruses can cause influenza-like illness during the year, influenza virus is usually the predominant cause of serious respiratory disease in a community.

Influenza A viruses are classified into subtypes based on their hemagglutinin (H) and neuraminidase (N) antigens. Recently circulating strains have possessed one of three H and one of two N antigens, and the subtypes are designated accordingly (e.g., H3N2, H1N1). Antibodies to these antigens, particularly to H antigen, can protect an individual against a virus carrying the same antigen. During inter-pandemic periods, minor H antigen changes ("drift") are common, and the greater the change the less will be the cross-immunity to the new strain conferred by the previously circulating virus. It is this antigenic variation from one influenza virus subtype to another that is responsible for continued outbreaks of influenza and necessitates annual reformulation of influenza vaccine. The antigens of influenza B viruses are much more stable than those of influenza A viruses and, although antigenic variation does occur, it is less frequent.

Pandemic influenza is usually associated with a major antigenic change or "shift" and the rapid global spread of influenza A virus having a different H and often a different N antigen from strains circulating previously. Canada, like other countries, has been affected by major influenza pandemics, e.g., in 1889-90 (H3N2), 1918-19 (H1N1), 1957-58 (H2N2) and 1968-69 (H2N2). Major epidemics of influenza A associated with smaller antigenic changes have also occurred.

Preparations Used for Immunization

Influenza virus vaccines available in Canada are inactivated suspensions of one or more strains of virus grown in hens' eggs with thimerosal as a preservative and possibly gelatin as a stabilizer. Tissue-culture derived vaccines and live attenuated vaccines are advanced in development.

The virus strains chosen for inclusion in influenza vaccine are reviewed annually to ensure that they include antigens that are expected to provide the best protection during the following winter. However, current vaccine production methods take at least 3.5 months, and are used in a batch process so that vaccine is available in early fall.

Vaccines are available as whole-virus or split-virus preparations. Split-virus preparations contain viruses that have been treated with an organic solvent to remove surface glycoproteins and thus reduce vaccine reactogenicity or capability to produce side effects. Split-virus and whole-virus vaccines are similar with respect to immunogenicity, but split-virus vaccine is generally associated with fewer side effects in children and young adults. *Only split-virus vaccines are recommended for use in people < 13 years of age. Vaccines are not approved for infants < 6 months of age.*

The effectiveness of influenza vaccine varies depending upon the age and immunocompetence of the vaccine recipient and the degree of similarity between the virus strain included in the vaccine and the strain of circulating virus during the influenza season. Over the last decade, improved global surveillance activities for influenza have resulted in the use of vaccine strains that are closely matched with circulating strains. With a good match, influenza vaccination has been shown to prevent illness in approximately 70% of healthy children and adults. Under these circumstances, studies have also shown influenza vaccination to be approximately 70% effective in preventing hospitalization for pneumonia and influenza among elderly persons living in the community. Studies among elderly persons residing in nursing homes have shown influenza vaccination to be 50% to 60% effective in preventing hospitalization and pneumonia, and up to 85% effective in preventing death, even though the efficacy in preventing influenza illness may often be in the range of 30% to 40%.

Storage requirements

The vaccine should be refrigerated at a temperature between 2° and 8° C. The vaccine should not be frozen.

Recommended Recipients

People at high risk

Vaccination of people at high risk is the single most important measure for reducing the impact of influenza. Priority should be given to ensuring annual vaccination of people in the following groups:

- Adults and children with chronic cardiac or pulmonary disorders (including bronchopulmonary dysplasia, cystic fibrosis and asthma) severe enough to require regular medical follow-up or hospital care. Chronic cardiac and pulmonary disorders are by far the most important risk factors for influenza-related death.

- People of any age who are residents of nursing homes and other chronic care facilities. Such residents often have one or more of the medical conditions outlined in the first group. In addition, their institutional environment may promote spread of the disease. Studies have shown that vaccinating staff members as well decreases the occurrence of illness and has an even greater impact on reducing the rates of hospital admission, pneumonia and death.

- People ≥ 65 years of age. The risk of severe illness and death related to influenza is moderately increased among healthy people in this age group, but is not as great as among those with chronic underlying disease. Vaccination is effective in preventing hospital admission and death.

- Adults and children with chronic conditions, such as diabetes mellitus and other metabolic diseases, cancer, immunodeficiency, immunosuppression, renal disease, anemia and hemoglobinopathy. The degree of risk associated with chronic renal and metabolic diseases is uncertain, but this uncertainty should not preclude consideration of vaccination.

- Children and adolescents (age 6 months to 18 years) with conditions treated for long periods with acetylsalicylic acid. This therapy might increase the risk of Reye syndrome after influenza.

- Persons infected with human immunodeficiency virus (HIV). There is limited information about the frequency and severity of influenza illness among HIV-infected persons, but reports suggest that for some the symptoms may be prolonged and the risk of complications increased. Because influenza can result in serious illness and complications, vaccination is a prudent precaution and will result in protective antibody levels in many recipients. However, the antibody response to vaccine may be low in persons with advanced HIV-related illnesses; giving a second dose of vaccine 4 or more weeks after the first does not improve their immune response. HIV load does not increase following influenza vaccination.

Influenza Vaccine

- People at high risk of influenza complications who are embarking on foreign travel to destinations where the virus is likely to be circulating should be vaccinated with the most current available vaccine. In the tropics, influenza can occur throughout the year; in the southern hemisphere, peak activity occurs from April through September, and in the northern hemisphere from November through March.

People capable of transmitting influenza to those at high risk

People who could transmit influenza to those at high risk should receive annual vaccination:

- Health care and other personnel who have significant contact with people in the high-risk groups previously described. A reduction in mortality and influenza-like illness was reported among patients in chronic care facilities when staff were also immunized. Every effort should be made to immunize both residents and staff in this setting.

- Household contacts (including children) of people at high risk who either cannot be vaccinated or may respond inadequately to vaccination. Because low antibody responses to influenza vaccine may occur in some people at high risk (e.g., the elderly, people with immunodeficiency), annual vaccination of their household contacts may reduce the risk of influenza exposure.

Other people

- Working adults. People who provide essential community services may be considered for vaccination to minimize the disruption of routine activities in epidemics. Other employers and their employees should consider yearly influenza vaccination for healthy working adults as this has been shown to decrease work absenteeism from respiratory and other illnesses and may be cost-saving.

- Pregnant women. Vaccination is recommended for pregnant women in high-risk groups. Influenza vaccine is considered safe for pregnant women at all stages of pregnancy.

- Travellers. Immunization may be considered for all individuals who wish to avoid influenza while travelling to areas where the virus is likely to be circulating.

Recommended Usage

One dose of either whole-virus or split-virus inactivated influenza vaccine is recommended for adults and children $\geq$ 13 years. Only split-virus vaccine is recommended for children < 13 years, in the dose recommended by the manufacturer. Previously unimmunized children < 9 years require two doses at an interval of 4 weeks; the second dose is not needed if the child received one or more doses of influenza vaccine prepared for a previous season.

Intramuscular (IM) administration is the preferred route, as data relating to influenza vaccine have generally been obtained after IM administration. The deltoid muscle is the recommended site in adults and older children, and the anterolateral thigh is recommended in infants and young children.

Protection generally begins about 2 weeks after injection and may last 6 months or longer. However, in the elderly, antibody levels fall below protective levels in 4 months or less. Thus, the preferred time for immunization of elderly individuals is November. Nevertheless, annual vaccination programs, such as those for residents of long-term care facilities, should begin as soon as vaccine is available in September or early October to ensure high coverage prior to significant virus circulation. Finally, no opportunity should be missed to give vaccine to an individual at risk who has not already been immunized for the current season, even if influenza activity has already started.

Table 1
Recommended Influenza Vaccine Dosage by Age

Age	Vaccine type	Dose (mL)	No. of doses*
≥ 13 years	Whole or split virus	0.5	1
9-12 years	Split virus	0.5	1
3-8 years	Split virus	0.5	1 or 2
6-35 months	Split virus	0.25	1 or 2

* Children < 9 years of age require two doses with an interval between doses of 4 weeks if the child did not receive at least one dose of influenza vaccine prepared for the previous season.

Adverse Reactions
Adults receiving the split-virus vaccine have shown no increase in the frequency of fever or other systemic symptoms compared with those receiving placebo. Fever, malaise and myalgia may occur within 1 or 2 days after vaccination, especially in young adults who have received the whole-virus vaccine and those receiving the vaccine for the first time.

In children aged 2 to 12 years given split-virus vaccine, fever and local reactions are no more frequent than after injection with placebo. In children < 24 months of age, fever occurs more often but is seldom severe.

Influenza immunization does not adversely affect the health of breast-feeding mothers or their infants.

Unlike the 1976-77 swine influenza vaccine, subsequent vaccines prepared from other virus strains have not been clearly associated with an increased frequency of Guillain-Barré syndrome. Influenza vaccine is not known to predispose to Reye syndrome.

Contraindications and Precautions

Influenza vaccine should not be given to individuals with known anaphylactic hypersensitivity to eggs manifested as hives, swelling of the mouth and throat, difficulty breathing, hypotension and shock. Allergic responses are rare and are probably a consequence of exquisite sensitivity to some vaccine component, most likely residual egg protein, which is present in minute quantities. Pregnancy and breast-feeding are not considered contraindications to influenza vaccination.

Simultaneous Administration of Other Vaccines

The target groups for influenza and pneumococcal vaccination overlap considerably. The concurrent administration of the two vaccines at different sites does not increase the risk of side effects. *Pneumococcal vaccine, however, is usually given only once, whereas influenza vaccine is given annually.* Children at high risk may receive influenza vaccine at the same time as routine pediatric vaccines but at a different site.

Strategies for Reducing the Impact of Influenza

Influenza immunization is the single most effective way of preventing or attenuating influenza for those at high risk of serious illness or death, and the rate of use of this vaccine in Canada has recently shown a marked increase. Influenza vaccine programs should aim to vaccinate at least 90% of eligible recipients. Nevertheless, only 70% of residents of long-term care facilities and 20-40% of adults and children with the medical conditions listed previously receive vaccine annually.

Strategies to increase overall coverage of the target groups can include the following:

- Educational efforts aimed at physicians and the public to address common concerns about vaccine effectiveness and adverse reactions. These concerns include the belief of patients at risk that they hardly ever get influenza, the fear of side effects from the vaccine, and doubt about its efficacy. **The advice of a health care provider is often a very important factor affecting whether a person seeks immunization**. Most people at high risk are already under medical care and should be vaccinated during regular fall visits.

- Standing-order policies in institutions allowing nurses to administer vaccine.

- Simultaneous immunization of staff and patients in nursing homes and chronic care facilities.

- Vaccination of people at high risk who are being discharged from hospital or visiting the emergency room in the autumn.

- Promotion of influenza vaccination in clinics that manage patients in high-risk groups (e.g., cancer clinics, cardiac clinics and pulmonary clinics).

- Use of influential health professionals as role models.

- Distribution of positive messages about the benefits and risks of immunization through community newspapers, flu information telephone numbers, and collaborating pharmacists and specialist physicians.

Indications for amantadine (see also current annual statement)

A further strategy for reducing the impact of influenza is amantadine prophylaxis. It is 70% to 90% effective in preventing illness caused by type A influenza viruses but is ineffective against type B strains. Amantadine prophylaxis should not replace annual influenza vaccination in groups for whom vaccine is recommended.

Amantadine may be used as follows:

1. For the control of influenza A outbreaks among high-risk residents of institutions.

2. As the sole agent for prophylaxis in people at high risk during an outbreak when vaccine is unavailable, contraindicated or unlikely to be effective because of a shift in the antigenic composition of the outbreak strain.

3. As an adjunct to late vaccination of people at high risk (continued for 2 weeks after appropriate vaccination is complete).

4. As a supplement to vaccination in people at high risk who are expected to have an impaired immune response to vaccine.

5. For unvaccinated people who provide home care for individuals at high risk during an outbreak (continued for 2 weeks after the care provider has been vaccinated).

Amantadine doses must be carefully calculated, taking into consideration the patient's age, weight, renal function and presence of other, underlying conditions. Any adjustments for renal function should be made in addition to adjustments for age. Careful monitoring for adverse reactions is important.

Influenza Vaccine

SELECTED REFERENCES

American Academy of Pediatrics Committee on Infectious Diseases. *The red book, report of the Committee on Infectious Diseases.* 24th ed. 1997. Elk Grove, Illinois: American Academy of Pediatrics, 1997:307-15.

Brown LE, Hampson AW, Webster RG, eds. *Options for the control of influenza III.* Amsterdam: Elsevier, 1996.

CDC. *Prevention and control of influenza: recommendations of the Immunization Practices Advisory Committee (ACIP).* MMWR 1995;44(No.RR-3):1-22.

Douglas RG Jr. *Prophylaxis and treatment of influenza.* N Engl J Med 1990;322:443-50.

Fedson DS. *Influenza and pneumococcal vaccination in Canada and the United States, 1980-1993: What can the two countries learn from each other?* Clin Infect Dis 1995;20:1371-76.

National Advisory Committee on Immunization (NACI). *Statement on influenza vaccination for the 1997-1998 season.* CCDR 1997;23(ACS-2):1-12.

Nichol KL, Lind A, Margolis KL et al. *The effectiveness of vaccination against influenza in healthy working adults.* N Engl J Med 1995;333:889-93.

JAPANESE ENCEPHALITIS VACCINE

Japanese encephalitis (JE) virus is the leading cause of viral encephalitis in Asia. Although 50,000 cases occur in Asia each year, infections have rarely been recognized in travellers. Countries where the disease occurs are listed in Table 1. The incidence of JE has been decreasing in China, Korea and Japan but increasing in Bangladesh, Burma, India, Nepal, Pakistan, northern Thailand and Vietnam.

Table 1
Countries Where Japanese Encephalitis Has
Been Recognized and Season of Epidemic Risk

Zone	Country
Temperate regions (Risk greatest in summer and autumn)	Bangladesh China Northern India Japan Kampuchea (Cambodia) Korea Laos Myanmar (Burma) Nepal Far Eastern Russia Northern Thailand Northern Vietnam
Tropical regions (Risk greatest during the rainy season)	Southern India Pakistan Indonesia Malaysia Philippines Sri Lanka Taiwan Southern Thailand Southern Vietnam

JE virus is an arthropod-borne flavivirus, a group that also includes yellow fever virus and St. Louis encephalitis virus. The main vectors are *Culex* mosquitoes, which breed mainly in rice fields. Swine and certain species of wild birds are intermediate hosts in the transmission cycle. Conditions that support the transmission cycle of JE virus are primarily rural agricultural ones, but occasionally cases are reported from urban areas. *Culex* mosquitoes tend to bite in the evening and night but day-biting species predominate in some regions.

Japanese Encephalitis Vaccine

The disease occurs in epidemic form in temperate and northern tropical regions and is endemic in southern tropical regions of Asia. Cases occur chiefly during the summer and autumn in temperate zones and during the rainy season in tropical zones. In areas where irrigation is the main factor affecting the abundance of vector mosquitoes, transmission may occur year round. For this reason, the periods of greatest risk for JE virus transmission to travellers are highly variable regionally and depend on such factors as season, location, duration of stay and the type of activities undertaken. Crude estimates for North Americans travelling to Asia place the overall risk of JE illness at less than 1 per 1 million. However, for persons travelling to rural areas during the transmission season, the risk per month of exposure is calculated to be 1 per 5,000.

Most JE infections do not result in obvious illness. Between 50 and 300 infections occur for each clinical case identified. Encephalitis, however, is usually severe, with a 10%-25% mortality rate and residual neuropsychiatric sequelae in 50% of cases.

The disease usually affects children, but in countries where it has been recently introduced all age groups may be affected. In addition to children < 10 years, an increased incidence has also been observed among the elderly in developed countries of Asia.

Limited data indicate that JE acquired during the first or second trimester of pregnancy causes intrauterine infection and miscarriage. Infections that occur during the third trimester of pregnancy have not been associated with adverse outcomes in newborns.

Since JE begins with an infected mosquito bite and < 3% of mosquitoes carry the virus, the risk for travellers can be significantly reduced by the appropriate use of bed-nets, repellants and protective clothing.

Preparation Used for Immunization

A highly purified formalin-inactivated vaccine derived from mouse brain has been licensed in Canada. The vaccine is produced by the Research Institute of Osaka University (Biken) and is distributed by Pasteur Mérieux Connaught (Canada). The vaccine contains thimerosal as a preservative.

This vaccine has been widely used in Asia. In Japan, where JE vaccine has been licensed since 1954, countrywide immunization for children was introduced between 1965 and 1968. In a study of children in Northern Thailand, the vaccine was demonstrated to have an efficacy of 91% (95% confidence interval 70%-97%). In this trial, immunization consisted of two subcutaneous 1.0 mL doses of vaccine, except in children < 3 years of age who received two 0.5 mL doses. A single dose of a similar vaccine was not found to have any efficacy.

Immunogenicity studies in the United States and Britain indicate that three doses are needed to provide protective levels of antibody in a suitable proportion of vaccinees. Less than 80% of vaccinees developed neutralizing antibody to two doses of vaccine, compared with 99% after three doses. After two doses of vaccine, antibody levels declined substantially in most vaccinees within 6 to 12 months (protective titres in < 29%). The response in Asian subjects after only two doses may reflect prior exposure to JE or other flaviviruses circulating in Asia. Although seroconversion rates are similar in Asian and non-Asian subjects who receive a primary series of immunizations over two weeks (day 0, 7, 14) or three weeks (day 0, 7, 30), the geometric mean titres are higher in the former group. The duration of protection after a complete primary series is unknown, but titres > 1:10 persist in 94% of healthy young adults for at least 3 years.

The lyophilized preparation should be stored at the temperature recommended by the manufacturer (2° to 8° C) until it is reconstituted with diluent. After reconstitution, the vaccine should be stored between 2° and 8° C and used within 8 hours.

Recent testing of a live-attenuated JE vaccine developed in China (SA14-14-2) suggests that this new product is both safe and efficacious. This vaccine may soon be widely available in Southeast Asia.

Recommended Usage

Vaccination is indicated for active immunization against JE for persons ≥ 1 year of age.

Vaccination is not recommended for all travellers to Asia. Vaccination should generally be considered for those who will spend 1 month or more in endemic or epidemic areas during the transmission season, especially if travel will include rural areas (see Table 1). However, there have been several reports of JE in short-term travellers to endemic regions. In special circumstances, vaccination should be considered for some persons spending less than 30 days in endemic areas, e.g., travellers to areas where there is an epidemic, travellers making repeated short trips, or persons with extensive outdoor rural exposure. *All travellers should be advised to take personal precautions against mosquito bites.*

Vaccination is recommended for all laboratory personnel working with JE.

A series of three 1.0 mL doses is given subcutaneously on days 0, 7 and 30. When time does not permit, they may be administered 5 to 7 days apart, but the response may not be as good.

Japanese Encephalitis Vaccine

113

Children 1 to 3 years of age should receive a smaller dose (0.5 mL) as directed by the manufacturer. There are no data on use of the vaccine in infants < 1 year of age. Wherever possible, immunization of infants should be deferred until they are 1 year of age.

No definitive recommendation can be made regarding the timing of boosters. In a study of 17 adults, elevated antibody titres persisted for 3 years after primary vaccination. No pediatric data are currently available. Booster doses of 1.0 mL (0.5 mL for children < 3 years) may be considered at intervals of 2-3 years.

Adverse Reactions

JE vaccine has been associated with injection site tenderness, redness and swelling. Other local effects have been reported in an average of 20% of vaccinees (range < 1% to 31%). Systemic side effects, principally fever, headache, malaise, rash and other reactions such as chills, dizziness, myalgia, nausea, vomiting and abdominal pain, were reported in about 10% of vaccinees. In an immunization program for U.S. military personnel in Okinawa, an overall reaction rate of 62.4 per 10,000 vaccinees occurred, including persons reporting urticaria, angioedema, generalized itching and wheezing. These reactions were generally mild to moderate in severity. Nine out of 35,253 persons immunized were hospitalized primarily to allow administration of intravenous steroids for refractory urticaria. None of these reactions was considered life threatening. A more recent study of 14,249 U.S. military personnel (36,850 doses of vaccine) demonstrated overall reaction rates of 16/10,000 for the first two doses and only 2/10,000 for the third dose. A history of any allergy (e.g., urticaria, allergic rhinitis, asthma) was associated with a slightly increased risk of reaction to JE vaccination.

Severe neurologic adverse effects such as encephalitis or encephalopathy have been reported after JE vaccination but are exceedingly rare (1-2.3 per million vaccinations).

Since 1989, an apparent increase in the incidence of hypersensitivity reactions in Canada, Denmark, Australia, the United Kingdom and Sweden has been reported, but the cause of these is unknown. The reactions are characterized by urticaria, often in a generalized distribution, and/or angiodema of the extremities, face and oropharynx, especially of the lips. Distress or collapse due to hypotension or other causes led to hospitalization in several cases. Most reactors have been treated successfully with antihistamines and/or oral steroids; however, some have had to be hospitalized for parenteral steroid therapy. Some reactors have complained of generalized itching without objective evidence of a rash. In the case-control study conducted as part of the JE immunization campaign in Okinawa it was found that persons developing these reactions after JE vaccination were more likely to have had a past history of urticaria after hymenoptera envenomation, drugs, or physical or other provocations, or urticaria of idiopathic origin.

An important feature of these reactions has been the interval between vaccination and onset of symptoms. Reactions after a first vaccine dose occurred after a median of 12 hours after vaccination; 88% of reactions occurred within 3 days. The interval between administration of a second dose and onset of symptoms generally was longer (median 3 days) and possibly as long as 2 weeks. Reactions have occurred after a second or third dose, when preceding doses were received uneventfully. Although some observers have reported that reactions occur chiefly after a second or third dose, one prospective study found similar reaction rates after first and second doses.

The vaccine constituents responsible for these adverse events have not been identified. Therefore, whether the rate of reaction to JE vaccine produced recently is associated only with certain lots or whether there is a uniform pattern that has gone undetected is uncertain.

Contraindications and Precautions

Allergic reactions to a previous dose of vaccine (generalized urticaria or angioedema) are contraindications to further doses. JE vaccine should not be given to persons with a hypersensitivity to proteins of rodent or neural origin or to thimerosal.

Epinephrine (1:1000) must be immediately available should an acute anaphylactic reaction occur due to any component of the vaccine.

Possible allergic reactions exhibited as generalized urticaria and angioedema may occur from minutes to as long as 9 days after immunization. Vaccinees should be observed for 30 minutes after immunization and warned against the possibility of delayed urticaria and angioedema of the head and airway.

Persons should not embark on international travel within 10 days of immunization because of the possibility of delayed allergic reactions and should be advised to remain in an area with ready access to medical care for 10 days after immunization.

A history of urticaria after hymenoptera envenomation, drugs, or physical or other provocations, or of urticaria of idiopathic cause should be considered when weighing risks and benefits of the vaccine for an individual patient. There are no data supporting the efficacy of prophylactic antihistamines or steroids in preventing JE vaccine-related allergic reactions.

The vaccine has not been assessed in pregnancy. It is not known whether JE vaccine can cause fetal harm when administered to a pregnant woman. Pregnant women who must travel to areas where the risk of JE infection is high should be vaccinated when the theoretic risks of immunization are outweighed by the risk of infection to the mother and developing fetus.

Japanese Encephalitis Vaccine

Persons undergoing immunosuppressive therapy may have a poor immunologic response to vaccines, and vaccination should be deferred, if possible, while patients are receiving such therapy. If travel must be undertaken, such patients may be immunized as already outlined with the understanding that the antibody response may be less than optimal.

There are no data on the effect of concurrent administration of other vaccines, drugs (e.g., chloroquine, mefloquine) or biologics on the safety and immunogenicity of JE vaccine.

SELECTED REFERENCES

Andersen MM, Ronne T. *Side-effects with Japanese encephalitis vaccine.* Lancet 1991;337:1044.

Berg SW, Mitchell BS, Hanson RK et al. *Systemic reactions in US Marine Corps personnel who received Japanese encephalitis vaccine.* Clin Infect Dis 1997;24:265-66.

CDC. *Inactivated Japanese encephalitis virus vaccine: recommendations of the Immunization Practices Advisory Committee (ACIP).* MMWR 1993; (No. RR-l):1-15.

Chambers TJ, Tsai TF, Pervikov Y, Monath TP. *Vaccine development against dengue and Japanese encephalitis: report of a World Health Organization meeting.* Vaccine 1997;15:1494.

Gambel JM, DeFraites R, Hoke C Jr, Brown A, Sanchez J, Karabastos N et al. *Japanese encephalitis vaccine: persistence of antibody up to 3 years after a three-dose regimen.* J Infect Dis 1995;171:1074.

Hoke CH, Nisalak A, Sangawhipa N et al. *Protection against Japanese encephalitis by inactivated vaccines.* N Engl J Med 1988;319:608-14.

Jelinek T, Northdurft HD. *Japanese encephalitis vaccine in travellers. Is wider use prudent?* Drug Safety 1997;16:153.

Liu Z-L, Hennessy S, Strom BL, Tsai TF, Wan C-M, Tang S-C et al. *Short-term safety of live attenuated Japanese encephalitis vaccine: results of a randomized trial with 26,239 subjects.* J Infect Dis 1997;176:1366.

Poland JD, Cropp CB, Craven RB et al. *Evaluation of the potency and safety of inactivated Japanese encephalitis vaccine in U.S. inhabitants.* J Infect Dis 1990;161:878-82.

Robinson HC, Russell ML, Csokoney WM. *Japanese encephalitis vaccine and adverse effects among travellers.* CDWR 1991;17:173-77.

Ruff TA, Eisen D, Fuller A et al. *Adverse reactions to Japanese encephalitis vaccine.* Lancet 1991;338:881-82.

Vaughn DW, Hoke CH. *The epidemiology of Japanese encephalitis: prospects for prevention.* Epidemiol Rev 1992;14:197-221.

Japanese Encephalitis Vaccine

MEASLES VACCINE

Measles (rubeola) is the most contagious vaccine-preventable infection of humans. There has been a marked reduction in incidence in countries where vaccine has been widely used, but measles remains a serious and common disease in many parts of the world. Complications such as otitis media and bronchopneumonia occur in about 10% of reported cases and are even more common in those who are poorly nourished and chronically ill, and in infants < 1 year of age. Measles encephalitis occurs in approximately 1 of every 1,000 reported cases and may result in permanent brain damage. In countries like Canada, death is estimated to occur once in 3,000 cases. Furthermore, prior measles infection is associated with subacute sclerosing panencephalitis (SSPE), a rare but fatal disease.

Because an effective vaccine is available and there is no non-human reservoir or source of infection, measles elimination within a population should be possible. During the XXIV Pan American Sanitary Conference in September 1994, representatives from Canada and other nations resolved to eliminate measles by the year 2000.

Before the introduction of the vaccine, measles occurred in cycles with an increasing incidence every 2 to 3 years. At that time, an estimated 300,000 to 400,000 cases occurred annually. Since the introduction of vaccine, the incidence has declined markedly in Canada (Figure 1). Only 203 cases were reported in 1993, the lowest ever recorded since notification began in 1924. Between 1989 and 1995, in spite of the very high vaccine coverage many large outbreaks occurred, involving mainly children who had received one dose of measles vaccine. It was estimated that about 10% of vaccinated children remained unprotected after a single dose given after 12 months of age. This proportion was large enough to allow circulation of the virus. To eliminate measles, it was thus necessary to change to a two-dose schedule to further decrease the proportion of susceptible children. In 1996 and 1997, every province and territory added a second dose to their routine schedule, and most conducted catch-up programs in school-aged children in order to protect those left susceptible after their first dose. These interventions achieved vaccine coverage for the second dose in excess of 85%, reducing the proportion of vulnerable children to a negligible level that will not sustain transmission of the virus. The great challenge for future years will be to continue administering two doses of vaccine to children as measles becomes increasingly unfamiliar to their parents.

In jurisdictions where programs are not achieving coverage rates of 95% or more with two doses, legislation could be considered that would require documented proof of immunization status as a prerequisite for entry to day care, school or university.

Figure 1: Measles - Reported Cases, Canada, 1924-1997

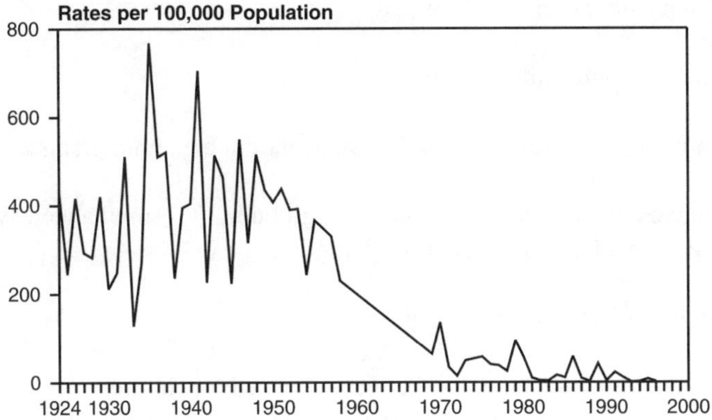

Rates per 100,000 Population

Measles live vaccine licensed in 1963
Measles killed vaccine licensed in 1964
Measles was not nationally reportable 1959-68

Preparations Used for Immunization

Live measles virus vaccines are prepared from Edmonston B "further attenuated" strains (e.g., Moraten, Edmonston-Zagreb, Schwarz, Connaught strains). They are available alone, in combination with live rubella vaccine (MR) or with mumps and rubella vaccines (MMR). Measles vaccines are generally prepared in chick fibroblast cell cultures, except for MoruViraten, which is grown in human fibroblasts. All preparations may contain traces of antibiotics (e.g., neomycin) and stabilizer such as gelatin. Consult the product monograph for details.

Recommended Usage
Children

For routine immunization, two doses of measles vaccine should be given. Infants should receive a first dose combined with mumps and rubella vaccines (MMR) shortly after their first birthday. The second dose should be given at least 1 month after the first, and before school entry. It is convenient to link this dose with other routinely scheduled vaccinations. Options include giving it with the next scheduled vaccination at 18 months of age, or with school-entry vaccinations at 4 to 6 years, or at any intervening age that is practicable (such as entry to day care). For routine second doses, MMR vaccine is preferred because a proportion of children will also derive protection against rubella and mumps. Measles-containing vaccine can be given concurrently with other childhood vaccines such as combined diphtheria, pertussis, tetanus, polio or *Haemophilus influenzae* type b vaccines. Separate injections are required in opposite anatomic sites.

Measles Vaccine

119

Two doses of vaccine given 1 month apart are recommended for children who

1. are out of step with the routine schedule;

2. are without an immunization record;

3. are without reliable records of measles immunization (e.g., immigrants);

4. were given live measles vaccine and immune globulin (IG) simultaneously or live measles vaccine within 5 months of receiving IG;

5. received an inadequate vaccine dosage.

Under certain conditions, vaccine may be recommended for children < 1 year of age. When an infant < 12 months of age is at high risk of exposure to measles or is travelling abroad to an area where measles is common, measles vaccine alone or as MMR may be given as early as 6 months of age. Under these circumstances, or if vaccine was inappropriately given before the child's first birthday, such children should receive two additional doses of MMR after the first birthday.

Susceptible persons > 12 months of age who are exposed to measles may be protected from disease if measles vaccine is given within 72 hours after exposure. There are no known adverse effects of vaccine given to persons incubating measles. However, IG given within 6 days after exposure can modify or prevent disease and may be used for this purpose in infants < 12 months of age, persons for whom vaccine is contraindicated or those for whom more than 72 hours but less than 1 week have elapsed since exposure (for IG dose see page 179). Unless contraindicated, individuals who receive IG should receive measles vaccine later, at the intervals specified in Table 7 on page 26.

Adults

Previously, routine vaccination was recommended for adults born after 1957. This cut-off has now been changed to 1970 because the recent epidemiology of measles in Canada has demonstrated that cases are very rare in adults born before that year. This observation is explained by the relatively free circulation of measles virus in Canada up until the early 1970s, allowing most people born before then to acquire measles. Although the vaccine was licensed for use in both Canada and the U.S. in 1963, it was used on a large scale in Canada only in the early 1970s, as compared with the mid 1960s in the U.S. Furthermore, in 1976, age at vaccination was raised to 15 months in the U.S. while it remained at 12 months in Canada. The greater proportion of primary vaccine failures associated with a younger age at vaccination permitted the large outbreaks of measles observed until the recent introduction of the two-dose schedule.

Measles Vaccine

A small proportion of adults born since 1970 are still vulnerable, and this proportion is greater among younger adults. Epidemiologic data show that settings with large concentrations of young adults, such as colleges and universities, permit transmission of measles. Thus, vaccine should be administered to adults born since 1970 who attend such institutions or who are expected to have a risk of measles exposure greater than among the general population (during travel or outbreaks). While two doses of vaccine or documented proof of disease are generally needed as evidence of complete protection, a single new dose of vaccine appears satisfactory to protect adults without such proof. In fact, most adults without proof of immunity are already immune, and a single dose of vaccine will raise that proportion close to 100%. The benefit of a second dose 1 month later is limited, because the largest cause of vaccine failure (anti-measles maternal antibody) is not a problem in adults. Second doses are recommended only for adults at greatest risk of exposure, as below.

One additional dose of vaccine should be offered to the following adults born since 1970 who have not already received two doses or suffered the disease:

■ Travellers to a measles endemic area

■ Health care workers

■ Students at post-secondary institutions

■ Military recruits

■ Adults who are aware that they were never immunized

Adverse Reactions

Measles vaccine produces a mild, non-transmissible and usually subclinical infection. Fever, with or without rash, may be seen in about 5% to 10% of persons 7 to 10 days after administration. Fever may occasionally trigger a seizure in susceptible individuals. Transient thrombocytopenia occurs rarely during the month after immunization. Adverse reactions are less frequent after the second dose of vaccine and tend to occur only in those not protected by the first dose.

Encephalitis has been reported in association with administration of live attenuated measles vaccine at a frequency of approximately 1 per million doses distributed in North America. Nevertheless, the reported incidence is much lower than that observed with the natural disease (approximately 1 per 1,000 cases).

The risk, if any, of SSPE developing after measles vaccination is considerably less than the risk after natural measles infection. No cases to date from whom measles virus was isolated had a vaccine strain. There has been a dramatic decline in the incidence of SSPE since the introduction of widespread measles immunization.

If MMR is used, reactions to the mumps and rubella components may be encountered (see pages 131 and 160).

Precautions and Contraindications

Administration of measles vaccine or MMR should be deferred with any severe acute illness. However, immunization should not be delayed because of minor acute illness, with or without fever.

Febrile seizures occasionally follow vaccination, particularly in children who have previously had convulsions or whose siblings or parents have a history of convulsions. However, the risk is low and the benefit of immunizing children greatly outweighs any potential risk associated with febrile seizures.

Tuberculosis may be exacerbated by natural measles infection, but there is no evidence that measles vaccine has such an effect. Measles vaccination can suppress a positive tuberculin skin test for several weeks. If skin testing for tuberculosis is required, it should be done on the same day as vaccination or delayed for 6 or more weeks.

Measles vaccine is specifically contraindicated in any individual whose immune system is impaired as a result of disease or therapy. However, MMR is indicated for most infants infected with the human immunodeficiency virus (HIV) whose immune function at 12 to 15 months of age is compatible with safe MMR vaccination (1994 Pediatric HIV Classification categories E, N1, A1). Consultation with an expert is required in the case of HIV-infected children to determine the presence or absence of significant immunodeficiency in individual cases. Measles revaccination may still be appropriate for HIV-infected persons with moderate immunodeficiency if there is a high risk of measles in the local community or travel to an area where measles is endemic. Consultation with local public health authorities will help determine the local level of measles activity and risk to travellers abroad.

Because the response to prior immunization may be impaired, HIV-infected children should receive IG after recognized exposures to measles. When other susceptible persons with immune deficiencies are exposed to measles, passive immunization with IG should be given as soon as possible (see page 179). It is desirable to immunize close contacts of immunocompromised individuals in order to minimize the risk of exposure of the latter to measles.

While there is no known risk from measles vaccine administered during pregnancy, it should not be given to pregnant women.

Egg allergy is no longer considered a contraindication to immunization with MMR. In persons who have a history of anaphylactic hypersensitivity to hens' eggs (urticaria, swelling of the mouth and throat, difficulty in breathing or hypotension), measles vaccination can be administered in the routine manner without prior skin testing. However, this should take place where adequate facilities are available to manage anaphylaxis. Persons at risk should be observed for 30 minutes after vaccination for any sign of allergic reaction. No special precautions are necessary for children with minor egg hypersensitivity who are able to ingest small quantities of egg uneventfully or who are given measles-rubella vaccine free of avian protein. No special measures are necessary in children who have never been fed eggs before MMR immunization. Prior egg ingestion should not be a prerequisite for MMR immunization.

Measles vaccine (or MMR) is contraindicated in individuals with a previous anaphylactic reaction to a measles-containing vaccine. If there is a compelling reason to re-immunize such individuals, MMR skin testing and graded challenge in an appropriately equipped facility can be considered. However, the possibility of a hypersensitivity reaction to the MMR skin test or during the graded challenge must be considered.

Since measles vaccine may contain trace amounts of neomycin, persons who have experienced anaphylactic reactions to topically or systemically administered neomycin should not receive measles vaccine.

For travellers, care must be taken in the timing of vaccination when IG is also required (see Table 7 page 26).

Outbreak Control

A full discussion of measles outbreak control is beyond the scope of this chapter. Readers are referred to the statement on outbreak control issued by the Advisory Committee on Epidemiology. With the current immunization coverage of two doses, large outbreaks of measles are not expected to recur. However, because many countries have lower immunization coverage, measles will continue to be imported into Canada. Imported cases will result in limited transmission of measles, usually occurring among unvaccinated children and young adults who have not received two doses of vaccine. As these outbreaks will die out by themselves, future efforts will be more productive if they are directed at maintaining high vaccine coverage in children rather than controlling sporadic outbreaks.

Control interventions in schools or other facilities had little impact when Canada was using a single dose program. With the two-dose strategy and high vaccine coverage, the benefits of control interventions are likely to be negligible except in settings where vaccine coverage is known to be low. Thus, before any intervention is started, suspected measles cases should be promptly confirmed by culture or serology. If cases are confirmed, contacts should be informed that measles is circulating and advised to update their vaccination status if necessary. For practical purposes, all students attending the same school or facility should be considered contacts. Immunization within 72 hours of exposure will usually prevent measles and is not known to produce adverse effects. Should an individual already be immune or infected by measles virus, there is no increased risk of adverse reactions from vaccination with live measles vaccine or with MMR.

Measles Vaccine

123

SELECTED REFERENCES

Advisory Committee on Epidemiology. *Guidelines for control of measles outbreaks in Canada.* CCDR 1995;21:189-95.

Bell A, King A, Pielak K, Fyfe M. *Epidemiology of measles outbreak in British Columbia — February 1997.* CCDR 1997;23:49-51.

De Serres G, Boulianne N, Meyer F, Ward BJ. *Measles vaccine efficacy during an outbreak in a highly vaccinated population: incremental increase in protection with age at vaccination up to 18 months.* Epidemiol Infect 1995;115:315-23.

Markowitz L, Albrecht P, Orenstein WA, Lett SM, Pugliese TJ, Farrell D. *Persistence of measles antibody after revaccination.* J Infect Dis 1992;166:205-08.

McLean ME, Walsh PJ, Carter AO, Lavigne PM. *Measles in Canada — 1989.* CCDR 1990;16:213-18.

Osterman JW, Melnychuk D. *Revaccination of children during school-based measles outbreaks: potential impact of a new policy recommendation.* Can Med Assoc J 1992;146: 929-36.

Ratnam S, Chandra R, Gadag V. *Maternal measles and rubella antibody levels and serologic response in infants immunized with MMRII vaccine at 12 months of age.* J Infect Dis 1993;168:1596-98.

Ratnam S, West R, Gadag V, Williams B, Oates E. *Immunity against measles in school aged children: implications for measles revaccination strategies.* Can J Public Health 1996;87:407-10.

Veit BC et al. *Serological response to measles revaccination in a highly immunized military dependent adolescent population.* J Adolesc Health 1991;12:273-8.

Wittler RR, Veit BC, McIntyre S, Schydlower M. *Measles revaccination response in a school-age population.* Pediatrics 1991; 88:1024-30.

Wong T, Lee-Han H, Bell B, Daley J, Bailey N, Vanderpol M. *Measles outbreak in Waterloo area, Ontario, 1990-1991.* CCDR 1991;17: 219-24.

Measles Vaccine

MENINGOCOCCAL VACCINE

The incidence of invasive meningococcal disease in Canada reached a peak of 1.6 cases per 100,000 population between 1989 and 1992. Since then, the number of cases has declined yearly, and the 1996 incidence of 0.9 per 100,000 (264 cases) was the lowest in 11 years. The meningococcal infection rate varies inversely with age. During 1996, children aged < 1 year had the highest age-specific incidence, of 11.1 per 100,000. Between 1993 and 1996 the case fatality rate steadily declined from 12.9% to 6.5%.

Sixty percent of all meningococcal isolates collected from cerebrospinal fluid and blood between 1992 and 1996 belonged to vaccine-preventable serogroups, including A, C, Y and W-135. Overall, the two most frequently isolated serogroups were C and B, accounting for 50% and 36% of laboratory-confirmed cases respectively. During this period, 90% of all serogroup C isolates belonged to a single clone (electrophoretic type ET15), which has been dominant in Canada since 1985.

Preparations Used for Immunization

Meningococcal vaccines contain purified capsular polysaccharides. Products available in Canada are a bivalent group A and C vaccine and a quadrivalent vaccine containing groups A, C, Y and W-135. No vaccine is licensed for use against group B strains.

Among adults and children ≥ 2 years of age, vaccines containing polysaccharides of groups A and C have generally been shown to be ≥ 90% effective in preventing meningococcal disease caused by the constituent groups during outbreaks in both civilian and military populations. A single dose is protective for at least 2 years. No cross protection occurs between serogroups.

In children aged 3 to 23 months, two doses of monovalent group A vaccine given 2 to 3 months apart have been shown to produce a high rate of seroconversion and to have a protective efficacy of 95% during disease outbreaks, with protection lasting for at least 1 year. In similarly aged children a single dose of group C vaccine produces an antibody response, but significant protective efficacy against group C disease has not been shown.

Children and adults produce an antibody response to vaccine containing polysaccharides of groups Y and W-135, but the degree of protection against disease has not been established.

Recommended Usage

Routine use of meningococcal vaccines for civilians is not recommended. For household contacts of sporadic cases of meningococcal disease, management should consist of chemoprophylaxis and close surveillance. The same recommendations apply for contacts who share sleeping arrangements with the index case, for child care and nursery school contacts, and for all people whose nose and mouth have been directly contaminated by oral or nasal secretions from someone with meningococcal disease.

Vaccination is recommended for selected individuals at increased risk of acquiring infection or of having fulminant disease, and for the control of outbreaks caused by the serogroups present in the vaccines. Vaccination is recommended for the following groups and situations.

1. Adults and children ≥ 2 years of age with functional or anatomic asplenia, because of the potential increased risk of fulminant meningococcemia. Whenever possible, vaccine should be given at least 10 to 14 days before splenectomy.

2. Populations clearly demonstrated to be at increased risk of infection, such as military recruits.

3. Outbreak control: the factors used to define an outbreak are addressed in the *Guidelines for Control of Meningococcal Disease* (1994). These factors allow identification of target groups to be included in a vaccination program on the basis of risk. The guidelines also include specific recommendations for the use of group C vaccine in outbreaks involving schools and other settings.

4. Individuals travelling to or living in an area outside of North America in which there is a high incidence of meningococcal disease. For updates on these areas consult a local travel clinic.

For individuals aged ≥ 2 years, a single dose of vaccine should be given. When there is a risk of exposure to group A disease, infants aged 3 to 23 months should receive two doses of vaccine given 2 to 3 months apart. When there is a risk of exposure to group C disease, infants aged 6 to 23 months may be given a single dose of vaccine, depending on the age-related occurrence of disease. Quadrivalent vaccine should be used unless the risk of exposure is known to be limited to a specific serogroup for which monovalent or bivalent vaccine is available.

Repeated Doses of Vaccine

The need for repeat doses of meningococcal vaccine and their optimal timing are unknown. The persistence of increased serum antibody concentration following group A or C vaccination is limited and age related. Among infants who have received two doses of group A vaccine, the antibody response persists for 1 year in those aged

126

< 12 months, and for 2 years in those aged 12 to 23 months. Among older individuals who have received a single dose of group A vaccine, the response persists for 2 to 3 years in those aged < 6 years, and for at least 5 years in older children and adults.

Unlike group A vaccine, a primary dose of group C vaccine does not prime the immune system for a booster response. However, for individuals immunized at ≥ 6 months of age, repeated doses do produce a significant increase in serum antibody concentration. For those immunized at ≤ 2 years of age, the response persists for only 6 to 12 months. Among older vaccinees the persistence may be for as long as 2 to 4 years.

Little is known about the duration of protection following administration of group Y and W-135 vaccine.

Until more information is available, additional doses of vaccine should be considered in the following situations:

1. **Group A disease**: If there is continued exposure during an outbreak or expected exposure as a result of travel to areas where the incidence of group A disease is high, the potential need for a repeat dose of vaccine depends on the age of immunization, the number of primary doses received and the interval since the last dose, as shown in Table 1.

Table 1
Indications for Repeat Doses of Vaccine against Group A Disease

Age when first immunized	No. of primary doses	Interval since last dose as indication for repeat dose
< 1 year	1 2	≥ 2 months 6-12 months
13-23 months	1	1-2 years
2-5 years	1	2-3 years
≥ 6 years	1	≥ 5 years

2. *Group C disease:* If there is continued exposure during an outbreak or expected exposure during travel to areas outside North America where the incidence of group C disease is high, a repeat dose of vaccine may be considered after 6 to 12 months for children first immunized at ≤ 2 years of age, and after 5 years for individuals first immunized after 2 years of age. Repeat dosing at 5 year intervals (or sooner in special circumstances) is recommended for individuals at increased risk of fulminant meningococcemia.

Adverse Reactions and Contraindications

Local redness, swelling and/or pain occur frequently, but these reactions are not severe and usually disappear within 1 to 2 days. Immediate wheal and flare reactions occur rarely. Systemic adverse reactions are uncommon and not severe. The incidence of adverse reactions is similar after a single and repeated doses of vaccine, provided the latter are given as recommended.

Pregnancy is not a contraindication to vaccination.

SELECTED REFERENCES

Ashton F, Ryan J, Borczyk A et al. *Emergence of a virulent clone of Neisseria meningitidis serotype 2a that is associated with meningococcal group C disease in Canada.* J Clin Microbiol 1991;29:2489-93.

Committee to Advise on Tropical Medicine and Travel (CATMAT). *Statement on meningococcal vaccination for travellers.* CCDR 1995;21:25-9.

Gold R, Lepow ML, Goldschneider I et al. *Kinetics of antibody production to group A and group C meningococcal polysaccharide vaccines during the first 6 years of life: prospects for routine immunization of infants and children.* J Infect Dis 1979;140:690-97.

King JW, MacDonald NE, Wells G et al. *Total and functional antibody response to a quadrivalent meningococcal polysaccharide vaccine among children.* J Pediatr 1996;128:196-202.

LCDC. *Guidelines for control of meningococcal disease.* CCDR 1994;20:17-27.

Lepow ML, Beeler J, Randolph M et al. *Reactogenicity and immunogenicity of a quadrivalent combined meningococcal polysaccharide vaccine in children.* J Infect Dis 1986;154:1033-36.

Peltola H, Makela PH, Kayhty J et al. *Clinical efficacy of meningococcus group A capsular polysaccharide vaccine in children three months to five years of age.* N Engl J Med 1977;297:686-91.

Reingold AL, Broome CV, Hightower AW et al. *Age-specific differences in duration of clinical protection after vaccination with meningococcal polysaccharide A vaccine.* Lancet 1985;2:114-18.

De Wals P, Dionne M, Douville-Fradet M et al. *Impact of a mass immunization campaign against serogroup C meningococcus in the province of Quebec, Canada.* Bull WHO 1996;74:407-11.

Whalen C, Hockin JC, Ryan A et al. *The changing epidemiology of invasive meningococcal disease in Canada, 1985 through 1992.* JAMA 1995;273:390-94.

Yergeau A, Alain L, Pless R et al. *Adverse events temporally associated with meningococcal vaccines.* Can Med Assoc J 1996;154:503-07.

Meningococcal Vaccine

MUMPS VACCINE

Mumps is an acute infectious disease caused by mumps virus. Subclinical infection is common. Although complications are relatively frequent, permanent sequelae are rare. Prior to widespread use of mumps vaccine, mumps was a major cause of viral meningitis. Transient but occasionally permanent deafness may occur, at an estimated rate of 0.5 to 5.0 per 100,000 reported mumps cases. Orchitis occurs in 20% to 30% of postpubertal male cases and oophoritis in 5% of postpubertal female cases. Involvement of the reproductive organs is commonly unilateral; therefore, sterility as a result of mumps is rare. Mumps infection during the first trimester of pregnancy may increase the rate of spontaneous abortion.

Since the introduction of vaccine, the incidence of clinical mumps has decreased by > 90% in Canada. Approximately 500 cases have been reported annually in recent years. Outbreaks are rare, but a localized one involving university students was reported in 1997. Mumps surveillance continues to be necessary to assess the effectiveness of immunization in children as well as adults.

Preparations Used for Immunization

Mumps virus vaccine is a live, attenuated virus vaccine and is available in combination with measles and rubella vaccines and in monovalent form. It is prepared from the Jeryl Lynn attenuated virus strain and is grown in chick embryo cell culture. A single dose of the vaccine produces an antibody response in over 95% of susceptible individuals. Antibody levels, though lower than those that follow natural disease, persist for at least 20 years and provide continuing protection. In a Canadian study, however, a significant proportion of the vaccinees were negative for mumps antibodies 5 to 6 years after immunization. There are no data currently available correlating specific antibody titres with susceptibility to mumps, but outbreaks have been reported in highly vaccinated populations. A two-dose measles-mumps-rubella vaccination schedule used in Finland resulted in higher mumps-specific antibody levels, higher seropositivity rate and slower decay of antibody levels.

Recommended Usage

Administration of live attenuated mumps vaccine in combination with measles and rubella vaccines (MMR) is recommended for all children ≥ 12 months of age. The combined vaccine should be used even in persons who may have prior immunity to components of the vaccine, and it can be used to immunize susceptible adults against mumps. Those considered susceptible are persons born in 1970 or later who have not had mumps (confirmed by a physician), have not been immunized, or do not present serologic evidence of immunity.

A universal second dose of mumps vaccine is conveniently achieved through a scheduled second MMR administration for children at 18 months or 4-6 years (refer to Tables 1, 2 and 3 of Immunization Schedules in Part 2).

Although mumps vaccination after exposure may not prevent the disease, it is not harmful. Should the exposure not result in an infection, the vaccine should confer protection against future exposures.

Adverse Reactions

Fever, parotitis and mild skin rashes may occasionally occur after vaccination. Very rarely, viral meningitis without sequelae has been reported. Only susceptible individuals are at risk for adverse reactions with second doses of vaccine.

Precautions and Contraindications

In common with other live vaccines, mumps vaccine should not be given to pregnant women or individuals whose immune mechanism is impaired as a result of disease, injury or treatment. An exception to this, however, is the recommendation that mumps vaccine, in the form of MMR, be given to HIV-infected children who are asymptomatic.

Mumps vaccine should not be administered less than 2 weeks before an immune globulin injection, or within 3 months after such an injection.

Convincing evidence supports the safety of routine administration of MMR vaccines to all children who have allergy to eggs. Refer to the Measles Vaccine chapter for further details.

Since mumps vaccine contains trace amounts of neomycin, persons who have experienced anaphylactic reactions to topically or systemically administered neomycin or to a previous dose of mumps-containing vaccine should not receive mumps vaccine.

SELECTED REFERENCES

Boulianne N, De Serres G, Ratnam S et al. *Measles, mumps and rubella antibodies in children 5-6 years after immunization: effect of vaccine type and age at vaccination.* Vaccine 1995;13:1611-16.

Cheek JE, Baron R, Atlas H et al. *Mumps outbreak in a highly vaccinated school population.* Arch Pediatr Adolesc Med 1995;149:774-78.

Davidkin I, Valle M, Julkunen I. *Persistence of anti-mumps virus antibodies after a two-dose MMR vaccination at nine-year follow-up.* Vaccine 1995;13:1617-22.

Griffin MR, Ray WA, Mortimer EA et al. *Risk of seizures after measles-mumps-rubella immunization.* Pediatrics 1991;88:881-85.

James JM, Burks AW, Roberson PK et al. *Safe administration of the measles vaccine to children allergic to eggs.* N Engl J Med 1995;332:1262-66.

Miller E, Goldacre M, Pugh S et al. *Risk of aseptic meningitis after measles, mumps and rubella vaccine in U.K. children.* Lancet 1993;341:979-82.

Peltola H, Heinonen OP, Valle M et al. *The elimination of indigenous measles, mumps and rubella from Finland by a 12 year two-dose vaccination program.* N Engl J Med 1994;331:1397-1402.

Mumps Vaccine

PERTUSSIS VACCINE

Pertussis (whooping cough) is a highly communicable infection of the respiratory tract caused by *Bordetella pertussis*. The disease can affect individuals of any age; however, severity is greatest among young infants. The goal of pertussis control is to reduce the incidence and severe morbidity of pertussis among young children. Pertussis has been controlled in Canada through immunization: during the last 40 years, the incidence of pertussis has decreased by > 90% (Figure 1), although outbreaks continue to occur. Over the past 10 years, the annual number of reported cases has ranged from 1,000 to 10,000 cases, although these figures likely under-represent the true incidence because of incomplete reporting. Hospitalization for pertussis is still common in Canada, and several deaths occur each year, particularly in unimmunized infants.

Figure 1: Pertussis - Reported Cases, Canada, 1924-1997

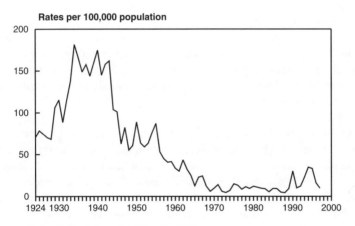

Rates per 100,000 population

Pertussis Vaccine was introduced in 1943

Preparations Used for Immunization
Whole-cell pertussis vaccines
Until recently, all pertussis vaccines available in Canada were so-called whole-cell vaccines, i.e., suspensions of killed *B. pertussis* organisms. With the licensure of acellular pertussis vaccines, which have better safety and efficacy profiles, the use of whole-cell pertussis vaccines is no longer recommended in Canada.

Acellular pertussis vaccines

Because of the frequency of local and systemic adverse reactions associated with whole-cell pertussis vaccines, acellular vaccines made from purified antigens of *B. pertussis* have been developed. All the currently available acellular vaccines contain pertussis toxoid (PT), and most contain filamentous hemagglutinin. Other antigens contained in some products are the 69 kilodalton (69 kDa) membrane protein, also known as pertactin, and fimbriae. Although just recently introduced into North America, acellular pertussis vaccines have been in widespread use in Japan for over 15 years.

Acellular pertussis vaccines are usually given combined with other agents, including diphtheria and tetanus toxoids (DTaP) with or without inactivated polio vaccine (DTaP-polio) and/or Hib conjugate vaccine (DTaP-Hib, DTaP-polio-Hib). Although not available at this time, combinations with hepatitis B vaccine are also under development.

Immunogenicity: There is no known direct correlation between serum levels of specific pertussis antibodies and protection against pertussis. A population's level of protection against pertussis correlates best with the presence of agglutinin antibodies, but these do not adequately predict protection in an individual. Acellular pertussis vaccines prepared from purified pertussis antigens evoke a predictable antibody response to all of the vaccine constituents. In comparative studies of these vaccines, however, the level of antibodies achieved after vaccination did not directly correlate with the antigen quantity in the vaccine.

Efficacy: In 1995-1996, the results of seven studies of the efficacy of eight DTaP vaccines were reported. The studies were not designed to compare the efficacy of acellular pertussis vaccines and involved different study designs; therefore, few conclusions can be drawn about the relative merits of the various products. All the acellular vaccines were efficacious; most were as effective or more effective than the whole-cell DPT vaccines included as a control condition. The duration of protection afforded by acellular pertussis vaccines is not known. Long-term follow-up is planned for several of the cohorts that participated in these efficacy studies. All acellular pertussis vaccines currently (1997) licensed in Canada have an estimated efficacy of approximately 85%; a detailed summary of the products and the results of the studies can be found in the 1997 NACI statement on acellular pertussis vaccines (see Selected References).

Storage requirements

Pertussis-containing vaccines should be stored between 2° and 8° C and should not be frozen. As with all adsorbed vaccines, pertussis-containing vaccines that have been frozen should not be used.

Recommended Usage

Vaccination against pertussis routinely consists of three doses given at 2, 4 and 6 months of age, a fourth dose at 18 months of age and a fifth dose at 4 to 6 years of age. When more rapid protection is preferred, the first three doses may be administered at intervals of 4 weeks and the fourth dose given as soon as 6 months after the third dose.

The dose should be as recommended by the manufacturer. All acellular pertussis vaccines are adsorbed vaccines and must be given intramuscularly. It is important that pertussis vaccination begin and be completed on time to ensure the greatest possible protection to the young infant, in whom the disease can be very serious.

Because adverse reactions may be more common and the disease is typically less severe in older children, adolescents and adults, immunization with the whole-cell pertussis vaccine was not previously recommended for persons ≥ 7 years of age. However, older children, adolescents and adults who develop pertussis are an important source of infection for young infants. For this reason, studies are under way to assess the role of pertussis in adolescents and adults with cough illness, and the safety, immunogenicity and efficacy of acellular pertussis vaccines in these age groups. Immunization in these age groups may be recommended in the future.

Acellular pertussis vaccine has been used safely for control of pertussis outbreaks in defined populations such as in schools or hospitals, although data supporting its effectiveness are lacking. Should its use be considered for this purpose, immunization with acellular pertussis vaccine should be undertaken with specific informed consent and with a formal evaluation of its effectiveness.

Although in 1998 whole-cell pertussis vaccine is still available, acellular pertussis vaccine is recommended for all children in Canada. For children who have already begun their immunization series with whole-cell pertussis vaccine, acellular vaccine should be substituted for the next and all subsequent doses. The efficacy of most of the acellular pertussis vaccines was demonstrated after three doses of the same vaccine; no data are available regarding the interchangeability of acellular pertussis vaccines. Therefore, whenever possible, efforts should be made to complete the first three doses with the same acellular vaccine. Although data are similarly lacking, the acellular vaccines can be considered interchangeable for the fourth and fifth doses because it may be difficult to ensure supply of the same vaccine during the entire 4- to 6-year immunization period.

Acellular pertussis vaccine is recommended to complete pertussis immunization in children whose series was interrupted because of the more extensive contraindications to pertussis immunization listed in previous editions of the *Canadian Immunization Guide* (see also "Conditions Not Considered Contraindications to Pertussis Vaccine"

Pertussis Vaccine

later in this chapter). Use of the acellular pertussis vaccine should also be encouraged for children from whose immunization series pertussis was removed because of false contraindications or parental concerns about adverse reactions associated with the whole-cell vaccine.

Vaccines that combine antigens against multiple diseases enhance immunization compliance by decreasing the necessary number of injections and visits, and therefore should be encouraged. Acellular pertussis vaccines are available as a pertussis-only vaccine and in combination with diphtheria and tetanus toxoids, as well as with inactivated polio vaccine and Hib conjugate vaccine. In general, adverse reactions associated with the combination vaccines are no more frequent than those associated with the constituent vaccines. Antibody responses to combination antigens are complex: combination vaccines may have increased, decreased or unaffected immunogenicity when compared with the individual vaccines, and the effects may differ among products from different manufacturers. As a rule, despite some "immune interference" between antigens, all licensed combination vaccines have demonstrated adequate immunogenicity with each of the constituent vaccines. For this reason, when combination vaccines are available, their use should be encouraged to facilitate compliance. Conversely, however, the need for multiple injections should not delay administration of vaccines that provide advantages of safety, immunogenicity, efficacy or cost.

Vaccines containing acellular pertussis may be administered simultaneously with other inactivated and live vaccines at different sites. None of the products should be mixed in the same syringe with any other vaccines unless specifically approved and described in the product monograph.

Children who have had natural pertussis can continue to receive pertussis-containing vaccines. Because of concern about adverse reactions associated with whole-cell pertussis vaccine, it was previously recommended that the pertussis component be removed from subsequent immunizations after a finding of positive pertussis culture, because of immunity conferred by infection. Although further data are needed, the increased safety profile of the acellular pertussis vaccine makes elimination of the pertussis component no longer necessary, and thereby simplifies immunization programs. As well, continuation of immunization with acellular pertussis vaccine may confer additional benefit to infants < 6 months of age, who often have a suboptimal antibody response to natural pertussis infection.

Adverse Reactions

The rate of reactions to acellular pertussis vaccines is less than that reported to whole-cell pertussis vaccines. In phase 2 and 3 studies of acellular pertussis vaccines the incidence rates of local adverse reactions, including tenderness, erythema, swelling and general reactions of fever, irritability and drowsiness, were significantly lower after immunization with acellular than with whole-cell pertussis vaccines. In a multicentre, phase 2 study sponsored by the U.S. National Institutes of Health, 13 acellular pertussis vaccines and two whole-cell pertussis vaccines were compared. Minor differences in rates of adverse events were demonstrated between the acellular vaccines, but none consistently resulted in fewer reactions. All were less likely than the whole-cell vaccines to lead to adverse reactions. In the large, phase 3 efficacy studies of acellular pertussis vaccines, less common adverse reactions such as persistent crying and hypotonic-hyporesponsive episodes were also less frequent after administration of acellular pertussis vaccines, and were reported in similar frequency among recipients of vaccines not containing pertussis. Convulsions were reported less often after immunization with acellular pertussis vaccines in some of the efficacy studies but not in others. Table 1 presents data from the Swedish efficacy study of two acellular pertussis vaccines, a U.S. whole-cell vaccine, and a diphtheria-tetanus toxoid vaccine (DT); these data are representative of rates of adverse reactions following pertussis vaccines.

Table 1
Adverse Reactions Associated with Pertussis Vaccine

Adverse reaction	Percentage reporting within 72 hours of one of three-dose infant series			
	DT (7,667 doses)	DPT (6,143 doses)	DTaP INFANRIX™* (7,650 doses)	DTaP (PENTACEL™) (7,699 doses)
Tenderness	22.20	80.50	21.80	22.20
Nodule ≥ 2 cm	6.00	22.30	6.60	7.80
Erythema ≥ 2 cm	3.50	14.60	3.10	4.80
Fever ≥ 38° C	34.80	90.40	35.20	36.90
Fever ≥ 40° C	0.09	0.46	0.05	0.03
Unusual cry	13.50	54.60	14.00	12.80
Persistent cry ≥ 1 hour	4.90	20.10	5.40	4.90
Persistent cry ≥ 3 hours	0.01	3.37	0.03	0.05
Convulsions	0.03	0.02	0.03	0.00
Hypotonic-hyporesponsive episode	0.00	0.08	0.00	0.01

* The INFANRIX™ in this study was a formulation that did not contain the 69 kDa.

Because of the lower incidence of fever associated with acellular pertussis vaccines, there may be less justification for routine use of prophylactic acetaminophen, as had been recommended with whole-cell pertussis vaccines. Acetaminophen may be considered in children with a high risk of febrile seizures or low pain tolerance.

Contraindications and Precautions

Pertussis vaccine should not be given to individuals who have had an anaphylactic reaction to a previous dose or to any constituent of the vaccine (see product monographs). Because these events are so rare, it is not known which component of the combined DPT or DTaP (or additional antigens in the combination vaccines) is responsible for allergic reactions. Therefore, no further doses of any of the vaccine components should be given unless assessment implicates the responsible antigen.

Conditions Not Considered Contraindications to Pertussis Vaccine

Certain other events temporally associated with whole-cell pertussis vaccination were at one time considered contraindications or precautions to further pertussis immunization. With the use of acellular pertussis vaccine, they are no longer considered contraindications.

- High fever within 48 hours of vaccination, attributed to vaccination and not to intercurrent illness, indicates the likelihood of recurrence of fever with subsequent doses. Febrile convulsions may be more likely in a susceptible child who develops high fever. However, there are no long-term sequelae from these convulsions, and pertussis vaccination can continue. Acetaminophen prophylaxis reduces the incidence of fever and may reduce febrile convulsions temporally related to pertussis vaccination.

- Afebrile convulsions have not been shown to be caused by pertussis vaccine and are not a contraindication to pertussis vaccination.

- Persistent, inconsolable crying and an unusual high-pitched cry after pertussis vaccination are not associated with any sequelae and are likely pain responses at the site of injection in young infants. These reactions do not preclude further pertussis vaccination. Acetaminophen prophylaxis may reduce discomfort with subsequent doses.

- Hypotonic-hyporesponsive episodes are not a contraindication to the use of acellular pertussis vaccine. Because these episodes occur after both DTaP and DT, it is difficult to attribute causation in recipients of DTaP to the pertussis component; continued immunization with all antigens is recommended.

- Onset of encephalopathy temporally related to pertussis vaccination does not indicate that the vaccine was the cause. Encephalopathy itself from whatever cause is not a contraindication to pertussis vaccination.

- Deferral of pertussis immunization for children with evolving neurologic conditions is no longer necessary because of the availability of acellular pertussis vaccines. Specific data on the use of these vaccines in individuals with neurologic diseases are not available and must await postmarketing surveillance. However, because the incidence of adverse events, including fever and seizures, was no different in recipients of DTaP and DT, it makes little sense to defer the pertussis component of the vaccine. Moreover, recent advances in the diagnosis and management of neurologic conditions leave little room for natural disease progressions to be misinterpreted as immunization-related events.

SELECTED REFERENCES

Information about specific products licensed in Canada can be found in the 1997 statement on acellular pertussis vaccines from NACI. This statement also lists unanswered questions about the use of acellular pertussis vaccines at the time of their licensure.

Decker MD, Edwards KM, Steinhoff MC et al. *Comparison of 13 acellular pertussis vaccines: adverse reactions*. Pediatrics 1995;96:557-66.

Edwards KM, Meade BD, Decker MD et al. *Comparison of 13 acellular pertussis vaccines: overview and serologic response*. Pediatrics 1995;96:548-57.

Edwards KM, Decker MD. *Acellular pertussis vaccines for infants*. N Engl J Med 1996;334:391-92.

Greco D, Salmaso S, Mastrantonio P et al. *A controlled trial of two acellular vaccines and one whole-cell vaccine against pertussis*. N Engl J Med 1996;334:341-48.

Gustafsson L, Hallander HO, Olin P et al. *A controlled trial of a two-component acellular, a five-component acellular, and a whole-cell pertussis vaccine*. N Engl J Med 1996;334:349-55.

National Advisory Committee on Immunization. *Statement on pertussis vaccine*. CCDR 1997;23(ACS-3):1-16.

Schmitt HJ, von Konig CHW, Neiss A et al. *Efficacy of acellular pertussis vaccine in early childhood after household exposure*. JAMA 1996;275:37-41.

Stehr K, Cherry JD, Heininger U et al. *A comparative efficacy trial in Germany in infants who received either the Lederle/Takeda acellular pertussis component DTP (DTaP) vaccine, the Lederle whole-cell component DTP vaccine, or DT vaccine*. Pediatrics 1998;101:1-11.

Trollfors B, Taranger J, Lagergard T et al. *A placebo-controlled trial of a pertussis-toxoid vaccine*. N Engl J Med 1995;333:1045-50.

Pertussis Vaccine

PNEUMOCOCCAL VACCINE

A polysaccharide vaccine is available against disease caused by 23 of the most common types of *Streptococcus pneumoniae* (pneumococcus). The overall incidence of invasive pneumococcal infections in Canada is not known precisely because the methods used to diagnose pneumococcal pneumonia are not very sensitive (blood culture) or specific (culture of sputum). In Canada, 16% of community-acquired pneumonia among adults has been attributed to pneumococcus. Invasive disease is most common in the very young, the elderly and certain specific groups at high risk. Data from the Canadian Sentinel Health Unit Surveillance System in 1996 show incidence rates of culture-proven invasive infection of 15/100,000 for all persons, 46/100,000 for persons $\geq$ 65 years of age, 23/100,000 for children 2-4 years old and 108/100,000 for children < 2 years old. The mortality rate due to pneumococcal pneumonia was 12.7% but it was 20.3% among those $\geq$ 65 years of age. Recent Canadian laboratory-based surveillance indicates that 7%-10% of the strains isolated from patients with invasive infection have reduced sensitivity to penicillin.

Preparations Used for Immunization

The current pneumococcal vaccine, available since December 1983, contains 25 µg of capsular polysaccharide from each of 23 types of pneumococci: 1, 2, 3, 4, 5, 6B, 7F, 8, 9N, 9V, 10A, 11A, 12F, 14, 15B, 17F, 18C, 19A, 19F, 20, 22F, 23F and 33F (Danish nomenclature). Approximately 90% of cases of pneumococcal bacteremia and meningitis are caused by these 23 types. The six serotypes that most often cause drug-resistant invasive pneumococcal infection are included in the vaccine. An earlier vaccine, which contained 50 µg of each of 14 types, was available between 1978 and 1983. The dose for all age groups is 0.5 mL, and vaccine may be given by either intramuscular or subcutaneous injection.

Available vaccines include Pneumovax 23 (Merck Frosst Canada), Pneumo 23 (Pasteur Mérieux Connaught Canada) and Pnu-Immune 23 (Wyeth Ayerst Laboratories). They contain the same serotype polysaccharides.

Effectiveness of the vaccine

In healthy young adults, a single dose of vaccine stimulates an antibody response to each of the component capsular polysaccharides. The immunity conferred is type specific. Efficacy, as measured by serotype-specific protection against invasive bacteremic pneumococcal disease, can surpass 80% among healthy young adults (evidence from randomized controlled trials), but is in the range of 50% to 80% among the elderly and specific patient groups, such as persons with diabetes mellitus, anatomic asplenia, congestive heart failure or chronic pulmonary disease (evidence from case-control and retrospective cohort studies). Antibody response and clinical

140

protection are decreased in certain groups at particularly high risk for pneumococcal infection. These include patients with renal failure, sickle-cell anemia or impaired immune responsiveness, including HIV infection. Response in children < 2 years of age is irregular and unsatisfactory. Following pneumococcal vaccination, serotype-specific antibody levels decline after 5 to 10 years and decrease more rapidly in some groups than others. The duration of immunity is not known precisely.

The results of economic analyses indicate that pneumococcal vaccine is cost-effective in the prevention of mortality and morbidity associated with invasive infections among persons at high risk and compares favourably with other standard preventive practices.

Recommended Usage

Pneumococcal vaccine is not recommended for children < 2 years of age because it is relatively ineffective. It is not recommended for the prevention of otitis media in childhood. Pneumococcal vaccine should be given to the following groups of adults and children > 2 years of age at increased risk of pneumococcal disease or its complications.

1. All persons ≥ 65 years of age. Pneumococcal vaccine may be administered simultaneously with influenza vaccine, at a separate anatomic site. Individuals with unknown vaccination histories should receive the vaccine.

2. All persons > 2 years of age with asplenia, splenic dysfunction or sickle-cell disease. Pneumococcal vaccine can be given simultaneously with Hib conjugate and meningococcal vaccines.

3. All persons > 2 years of age with the following conditions: chronic cardiorespiratory disease (except asthma), cirrhosis, alcoholism, chronic renal disease, nephrotic syndrome, diabetes mellitus, chronic cerebrospinal fluid leak, HIV infection and other conditions associated with immunosuppression (Hodgkin's disease, lymphoma, multiple myeloma, induced immunosuppression for organ transplantation).

Immunologic abnormalities may decrease both the antibody response to and protection by vaccine. When possible, vaccine should be given at least 10 to 14 days before splenectomy or initiation of immunosuppression therapy and early in the course of HIV infection. Because of variable vaccine efficacy in certain groups, those at highest risk (and their families) should be counselled regarding fulminant pneumococcal sepsis, which may occur despite vaccination. In these highest risk patients, some authorities recommend continuous antimicrobial prophylaxis. Measurement of antibody responses is not recommended because results are not readily obtained or interpreted.

Pneumococcal Vaccine

141

Revaccination

Results from serologic and case-control studies indicate that vaccine-induced immunity decreases with time. At present, routine revaccination is not recommended but revaccination should be considered for those of any age at highest risk of invasive infection as detailed below. Experience with revaccination is still limited, and there are no data on the relative effectiveness of a second dose.

Persons for whom revaccination should be considered include those with functional or anatomic asplenia or sickle-cell disease; debilitating cardiorespiratory disease; hepatic cirrhosis; chronic renal failure or nephrotic syndrome; HIV infection; and immunosuppression related to disease or therapy.

A single revaccination is recommended after 5 years in those aged > 10 years and after 3 years in those aged ≤ 10 years at the time of revaccination. Any need for subsequent doses remains to be determined.

Adverse Reactions

Reactions to vaccine are usually mild. Local soreness and erythema are quite common. Occasionally, slight fever may occur. Studies involving immunocompetent individuals showed that revaccination less than 2 years after an initial dose increased local and systemic reactions. Local reactions of the Arthus type have been observed rarely and may be severe. When revaccination is done after an interval of 3 years or more, the rate of adverse reactions is not greater than the rate after a first dose.

Precautions and Contraindications

Anaphylactic reaction to pneumococcal vaccine is a contraindication to revaccination. Pregnancy is not a contraindication to pneumococcal vaccine.

Strategies to Improve Vaccine Utilization

Vaccination is a safe and effective means of preventing invasive pneumococcal infection in groups at increased risk of serious illness or death. It offers a partial solution to the problem of emerging antibiotic resistance among pneumococci. However, recent surveys show that fewer than 5% of the population at increased risk have received this vaccine. Several provinces have initiated programs to make pneumococcal vaccine more readily available to target populations.

At a Canadian Consensus Conference on Preventing Pneumococcal Disease, held early in 1998, delegates concluded that the evidence strongly supports inclusion of pneumococcal vaccine in publicly funded immunization programs in all provinces and territories. Delegates considered that 40% reductions in the incidence of invasive pneumococcal infections and associated mortality rates were feasible by the year 2005 with effective immunization programs that were able to include 80% or more of those at high risk. A number of innovative strategies will be needed to meet these targets.

Recommended strategies for delivering pneumococcal vaccine include:

- Ensuring that all recipients of influenza vaccine are also appropriately immunized with pneumococcal vaccine, if eligible. Providers should have both vaccines available to facilitate their concurrent administration.

- Implementing standing orders for pneumococcal vaccination of residents on admission to long-term care facilities.

- Implementing standing orders in hospitals for pneumococcal vaccination of persons in high-risk groups to be vaccinated on discharge or during ambulatory visits.

- Delivering pneumococcal vaccine in adult day care and community centres to persons at risk.

- Promoting pneumococcal and influenza vaccination programs concurrently, to both consumers and providers.

SELECTED REFERENCES

Butler JC, Breiman RF, Campbell JF et al. *Pneumococcal polysaccharide vaccine efficacy: an evaluation of current recommendations.* JAMA 1993; 270:1826-31.

Fedson DS. *Clinical practice and public policy for influenza and pneumococcal vaccination of the elderly.* Clin Geriatr Med 1992;8:183-99.

Fine MJ, Smith MA, Carson CA et al. *Efficacy of pneumococcal vaccination in adults: a meta-analysis of randomized controlled trials.* Arch Intern Med 1994;154:2666-77.

Fine MF, Smith MA, Carson CA et al. *Prognosis and outcome of patients with community-acquired pneumonia. A meta-analysis.* JAMA 1996;275:134-41.

Gable CB, Holzer SS, Engelhart L et al. *Pneumococcal vaccine: efficacy and associated cost savings.* JAMA 1990;264:2910-15.

Marrie TJ Durant H, Yates L. *Community-acquired pneumonia requiring hospitalization: 5-year prospective study.* Rev Infect Dis 1989;11:586-99.

Rodriguez R. *Safety of pneumococcal revaccination.* J Gen Intern Med 1995;10:511-2.

Shapiro ED, Berg AT, Austrian R et al. *The protective efficacy of polyvalent pneumococcal polysaccharide vaccine.* N Engl J Med 1991;325:1453-60.

Snow R, Babish JD, McBean AM. *Is there any connection between a second pneumonia shot and hospitalization among Medicare beneficiaries?* Public Health Rep 1995;110:720-25.

Pneumococcal Vaccine

POLIOMYELITIS VACCINE

Poliomyelitis is a highly infectious disease caused by one of three types of the enterovirus poliovirus. It is extremely stable and can remain viable in the environment for long periods of time. The last major epidemic occurred in 1959, when there were 1,887 paralytic cases. Following the introduction of inactivated poliovirus vaccines (IPV) in Canada in 1955 and of trivalent oral poliovirus vaccine (OPV) in 1962, the indigenous disease has been eliminated (Figure 1).

Figure 1: Poliomyelitis, Paralytic - Reported Cases, Canada, 1949-97

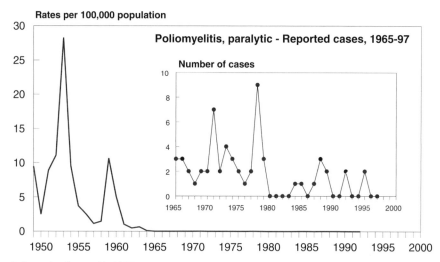

Salk vaccine licensed in 1955
Sabin vaccine licensed in 1962

The last significant outbreak occurred in 1978-79, when there were 11 cases of paralytic disease among unimmunized contacts of imported cases in religious groups in Ontario, Alberta and British Columbia. In 1993, 22 asymptomatic cases of imported wild polio infection were documented in the same religious group in Alberta. In addition, an importation of wild virus was documented in an asymptomatic child in Ontario in 1996. In none of these instances was spread of the virus seen outside the unimmunized groups, presumably because of high levels of immunization in the rest of the population.

Since 1980, 12 paralytic cases have been reported in Canada, 11 of which were determined to be vaccine-associated paralytic poliomyelitis (VAPP). Since 1987, all suspected cases of paralytic poliomyelitis have been reviewed by a subcommittee of

NACI or, since 1994, the National Working Group on Polio Eradication. The last reported case caused by a wild poliovirus occurred in 1988 and was found to be due to an imported strain from the Indian subcontinent. Of the other 11 cases, three have been classified as "confirmed" vaccine-associated contact cases, five as "possible" vaccine-associated contact cases and one as a "confirmed" vaccine-associated recipient case. Two other reported cases were not reviewed but occurred in known contacts of OPV-vaccinated children. The last reported case of VAPP occurred in 1995.

In 1985, the Pan-American Health Organization adopted a goal of elimination of poliomyelitis from the hemisphere, and this goal was achieved by September 1995. WHO adopted a similar goal, of global elimination, by the year 2000.

Preparations Used for Immunization

Both inactivated (IPV) and live oral (OPV) poliovirus vaccines are licensed for use, but because of the epidemiologic pattern only IPV is recommended for routine use in Canada. OPV is not discussed in detail in this chapter, and readers interested in more information about it are referred to earlier editions of the Guide.

There are two IPV preparations, one produced on Vero cells and the other on human diploid (MRC-5) cells. Both are formalin-inactivated products with enhanced potency and are significantly more immunogenic than the original IPV. They each contain the three types of wild poliovirus. A separate polio vaccine as well as combination products containing DPT or DTaP and IPV are available.

IPV is injected subcutaneously according to the dose specified in the manufacturer's package insert. Combination vaccines must be administered intramuscularly because of the presence of adsorbed tetanus and diphtheria toxoids. IPV produces immunity to all three types of poliovirus in over 90% of persons following two doses of vaccine given at least 6 weeks apart, and in close to 100% following a booster given 6 to 12 months later. The immune response induced in IPV vaccinees reduces the degree and duration of pharyngeal and fecal excretion of poliovirus after OPV challenge, as compared with unvaccinated children. However, IPV produces less mucosal immunity than OPV.

Recommended Usage

Infants and children

To avoid the risk of VAPP, exclusive use of IPV is recommended in Canada. Use of OPV alone or sequential use of IPV followed by OPV provides acceptable levels of protection but both carry the risk of VAPP in recipients or their contacts. Two doses of IPV are recommended 6 to 8 weeks apart, followed by a booster dose 6 to 12 months later. When given combined with DPT (or DTaP), it is acceptable to give additional doses of IPV 4 to 6 weeks after the second dose and 36 to 56 months after the booster dose for convenience of administration.

Children who began their polio immunization series in a jurisdiction where OPV is used may continue their immunization using IPV. There is no need to restart the series.

Adults

Routine immunization against poliomyelitis of adults living in Canada is not considered necessary. Most adults are already immune and have a very low risk of exposure to wild polioviruses in North America.

Primary immunization with poliomyelitis vaccine is recommended, however, for certain categories of adults who are at greater risk of exposure to poliovirus than the general population. Such persons include the following:

1. travellers to areas of countries where poliomyelitis is epidemic or endemic;

2. laboratory workers handling specimens that may contain polioviruses;

3. health care workers in close contact with individuals who may be excreting wild or vaccine strains of polioviruses; and

4. unvaccinated parents or child care workers who will be caring for children in jurisdictions where OPV is used.

In the case of these categories, the following recommendations apply.

A. *For unvaccinated adults*, primary immunization with IPV is recommended as two doses given at an interval of 1 to 2 months with a further dose 6 months to 1 year later.

Travellers who will be departing in < 4 weeks should receive a single dose of IPV and the remaining doses later, at the recommended intervals.

In unvaccinated parents or other household contacts of infants who are to be given OPV there is a very small risk of OPV-associated paralysis developing. It will generally not be practical for such persons to be fully protected with IPV before the infant is vaccinated, and the risk may be reduced by giving them one dose of IPV at the same time as the first dose is given to the infant. Arrangements should be made for the adults to complete their basic course of immunization.

B. *Incompletely immunized adults* who have previously received less than a full primary course of IPV or OPV should receive the remaining dose(s) of poliovirus vaccine as IPV, regardless of the interval since the last dose.

146

Booster doses for adults

The need for booster doses of poliovirus vaccine in fully vaccinated adults has not been established. Booster doses of vaccine are not routinely recommended for travellers, but a single booster dose of IPV (or OPV) might be considered for persons believed to be at greatly increased risk of exposure (e.g., the military, workers in refugee camps in endemic areas).

Outbreak Control

If transmission of paralytic poliomyelitis caused by wild virus occurs in a community, OPV should be administered to all individuals (including infants) who have not been completely immunized or whose immunization status is uncertain.

IPV is not recommended for the control of outbreaks of poliomyelitis.

Adverse Reactions

Individuals travelling or living abroad and whose children may be exposed to OPV should be aware that OPV may cause paralytic disease (see previous editions of the Guide).

The side effects of currently available IPV are limited to minor local reactions.

Precautions and Contraindications

IPV should not be administered to persons who have experienced an anaphylactic reaction to a previous dose of IPV, streptomycin, polymyxin B or neomycin.

IPV can be given without risk to those who are immunodeficient or immunosuppressed or to persons who will have household or similarly close contact with such persons. Less than optimal protection may be induced in those who are immunocompromised.

IPV is not contraindicated in pregnancy but, as for all agents, its administration should be delayed until after the first trimester if possible. IPV is always the vaccine of choice except for outbreak control.

Poliomyelitis Vaccine

SELECTED REFERENCES

American Academy of Pediatrics. *Poliomyelitis prevention: recommendations for use of inactivated poliovirus vaccine and live oral poliovirus vaccine.* Pediatrics 1997;99:300-05.

Cochi SL, Hull HF, Sutter RW et al. *Commentary: the unfolding story of global poliomyelitis eradication.* J Infect Dis 1997;175(Suppl. 1):S1-3.

Duclos P. *Paralytic poliomyelitis eradication: when success and forgetting may mean danger.* Can J Infect Dis 1992;3:142-43.

Hull HF, Birmingham ME, Melgaard B et al. *Progress toward global polio eradication.* J Infect Dis 1997;175(Suppl. 1):S4-9.

Kimpen JLL, Ogra PL. *Poliovirus vaccines: a continuing challenge.* Pediatr Clin N Am 1990;37:627-47.

Melnick JL. *Poliomyelitis: eradication in sight.* Epidemiol Infect 1992;108:1-18.

Modlin JF, Halsey NA, Thomas ML et al. *Humoral and mucosal immunity in infants induced by three sequential inactivated poliovirus vaccine-live attenuated oral poliovirus vaccine immunization schedules.* J Infect Dis 1997;175(Suppl. 1):S228-34.

Sabin AB. *My last will and testament on rapid elimination and ultimate global eradication of poliomyelitis and measles.* Pediatrics 1992;90:162-69.

Strebel PM, Sutter RW, Cochi SL et al. *Epidemiology of poliomyelitis in the United States one decade after the last reported case of indigenous wild-virus associated disease.* Clin Infect Dis 1992;14:568-79.

Vidor E, Meschievitz C, Plotkin S. *Fifteen years of experience with Vero-produced enhanced potency inactivated poliovirus vaccine.* Pediatr Infect Dis J 1997;16:312-22.

Wright PF, Kim-Farley RJ, de Quadros CA et al. *Strategies for the global eradication of poliomyelitis by the year 2000.* N Engl J Med 1991;325:1774-79.

RABIES VACCINE

Rabies virus can infect any mammal. In North America, it occurs mainly in certain wildlife species and is spread by them to domestic livestock and pets. In recent years, most reported wildlife infections in British Columbia have been in bats; in Alberta, Saskatchewan and Manitoba in skunks; in Ontario and Quebec in foxes and skunks; and in the Northwest Territories in foxes. Rabies has been reported sporadically from New Brunswick and Nova Scotia, and recently outbreaks in foxes have been reported in Labrador. Bat rabies is found in all regions across Canada and in most of the larger islands as far north as bats are found. Although infections in domestic dogs and cats account for less than 10% of reported animal rabies, the bites of these species account for the vast majority of suspected rabies exposures in humans and thus the majority of courses of post-exposure rabies prophylaxis.

Since reporting began in 1925, 21 persons have died of rabies in Canada (Figure 1). Even though disease may not develop in everyone bitten by a rabid animal, a decision on the management of a person who may have been exposed to rabies virus must be made rapidly and judiciously since delay in starting post-exposure prophylaxis reduces its effectiveness. It has been estimated that the risk of rabies developing if post-exposure prophylaxis is not given ranges from 3%-10% after a bite on the lower leg by a rabid dog to 50%-80% after multiple bites to the face and head by a rabid wolf. Since it is not possible to distinguish between those in whom rabies will or will

Figure 1: Rabies - Number of Deaths, Canada, 1924-1997

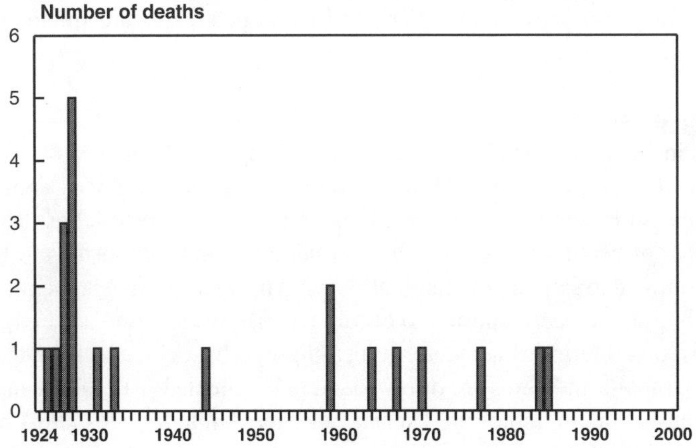

not develop if untreated and since the infection is almost always fatal, it is essential that all persons exposed to proved or suspected rabid animals be given post-exposure prophylaxis. Between 1,000 and 1,500 persons in Canada receive post-exposure treatment each year because of exposure to rabid or suspected rabid animals.

Among recent human cases in the U.S., infections with bat rabies virus strains have predominated, the problem being failure to recognize the small wound inflicted by a biting bat and thus omission of post-exposure prophylaxis.

Preparations Used for Immunization

Two rabies vaccines for use in humans are licensed in Canada: Imovax® rabies and Rabies Vaccine Inactivated (Diploid Cell Origin)-Dried. Both products are available from Pasteur Mérieux Connaught. Both may be used for pre-exposure and post-exposure prophylaxis and are administered by intramuscular injection. Both are prepared from rabies virus grown in human diploid cell culture and inactivated with beta-propiolactone. Human diploid cell vaccine (HDCV) together with rabies immune globulin (RIG) and local treatment is highly effective in preventing rabies in exposed individuals. No post-exposure HDCV failures have occurred in Canada or the United States. The few reported failures elsewhere have been attributed to delay in treatment, lack of appropriate cleansing of wounds, suboptimal methods of vaccination (in particular failure to administer vaccine into the deltoid muscle) or omission of passive immunization. Responses to vaccines produced in other countries may be less predictable.

Post-Exposure Management

Rabies prophylaxis must be considered in every incident in which potential exposure to rabies virus has occurred, unless rabies is known to be absent from the animal population. In evaluating each case, local public health officials should be consulted. If there has been no exposure as described below, post-exposure treatment is not indicated.

1. Species of animal

The animals in Canada most often proven rabid are foxes, skunks, cattle, dogs, cats and bats. The distribution of animal rabies and the species involved vary considerably across Canada, so in cases of possible exposure it is important to consult the local medical officer of health or government veterinarian. Human exposures to livestock are usually confined to salivary contamination, with the exception of horses and swine, from which bites have been reported to occur. The risk of infection after exposure to rabid cattle is low. Squirrels, hamsters, guinea-pigs, gerbils, chipmunks, rats, mice or other rodents, rabbits and hares are rarely found to be infected with rabies and are not known to cause human rabies in Canada and the United States. Post-exposure prophylaxis should be considered if the animal's behaviour was highly unusual.

The manifestations of rabies and the incubation periods vary in different species. The length of time virus may be excreted in saliva before the development of symptoms has not been determined for the purpose of defining rabies exposure except in dogs and cats. In these two species, rabies virus excretion does not generally precede symptom development beyond 10 days.

2. Type of exposure

Rabies is transmitted when the virus is inoculated into tissues, most commonly when virus in saliva is introduced into tissues by bites. Transmission can also occur when cuts or wounds of skin or mucous membranes are contaminated with virus in saliva or infected tissues. Rarely, transmission has been recorded when virus was inhaled, or infected corneal grafts were transplanted into patients. Thus, two broad categories of exposure are recognized as warranting post-exposure prophylaxis:

Bite: any penetration of skin by teeth. Bites inflicted by most animals are readily apparent. However, bites inflicted by bats to a sleeping person may not be felt, and these animals' needle-like teeth may leave no visible bite marks. Hence, when persons are sleeping unattended in a room where a bat is present and they cannot reasonably exclude the possibility of a bite, post-exposure prophylaxis should be initiated.

Non-bite: includes contamination of scratches, abrasions or cuts of skin or mucous membranes by saliva or other potentially infectious material, such as the brain tissue of a rabid animal. Petting a rabid animal or handling its blood, urine or feces is not considered to be exposure nor is being sprayed by a skunk. Such incidents do not warrant post-exposure prophylaxis.

Post-exposure prophylaxis is warranted and recommended in rare instances of non-bite exposure, such as inhalation of aerosolized virus by spelunkers exploring caves inhabited by infected bats or by laboratory technicians homogenizing tissues infected with rabies virus; however, the efficacy of prophylaxis after such exposures is unknown. Stringent guidelines concerning the suitability of tissue donors have eliminated the probability that rabies virus will be transmitted iatrogenically.

Non-bite (and bite) exposures incurred in the course of caring for humans with rabies could theoretically transmit the infection. No case of rabies acquired in this way has been documented, but post-exposure prophylaxis should be considered for exposed individuals.

3. Investigation of the incident

Each incident of possible exposure requires full investigation, including an assessment of the risk of rabies in the animal species involved and the behaviour of the particular animal. An unprovoked attack is more apt to indicate that the animal is rabid. Nevertheless, rabid cats and dogs may become uncharacteristically quiet. Bites inflicted on a person attempting to feed or handle an apparently healthy animal should generally be regarded as provoked.

A small number of animals have developed rabies despite prior vaccination. Therefore, even vaccinated animals must be carefully evaluated if they are exhibiting signs suggesting rabies. The vaccination history in itself should not influence the need for post-exposure treatment or the need to sacrifice the animal for assessment.

Management of Animals Involved in Biting Incidents

Any animal that has bitten a human or is suspected of being rabid should be reported to the local medical officer of health and to the nearest Canadian Food Inspection Agency veterinarian.[1] These veterinarians are familiar with the regulations concerning rabies and, if necessary, will collect and ship appropriate specimens to a federal laboratory for diagnosis.

Signs of rabies cannot be reliably interpreted in wild animals. These animals, as well as stray or unwanted dogs or cats and other biting animals, should be humanely killed immediately in a way that does as little damage as possible to the head, which should be submitted for laboratory examination. A domestic dog or cat that is evaluated as normal by a veterinarian should be kept under secure observation for 10 days even if it has a history of vaccination. If the animal is still clinically well after that time, it can be concluded that it was not shedding rabies virus at the time of the exposure incident and was therefore non-infectious. If illness suggestive of rabies develops during the holding period, the animal should be killed and the head submitted for examination. Rabies virus is only readily demonstrable in brains of animals that have neurologic symptoms. If the animal escapes during the 10-day observation period, the need for post-exposure prophylaxis should be carefully reassessed. Exotic pets (including ferrets) should be treated as wild animals because the incubation period and period of rabies shedding in these animals are unknown.

Management of Persons Following Possible Exposure to Rabies (Table 1)

The following recommendations are intended as a guide and may need to be modified in accordance with the specific circumstances of the exposure to rabies.

Local treatment of wounds

Immediate washing and flushing with soap and water, detergent or water alone is imperative and is probably the most effective procedure in the prevention of rabies. Suturing of the wound should be avoided if possible. Tetanus prophylaxis and antibacterial drugs should be given as required.

---

[1]   Further information and advice is obtainable from the Canadian Food Inspection Agency regional offices in Moncton, N.B. (506) 851-7651; Montreal, Que. (514) 283-8888; Guelph, Ont. (519) 837-9400; Winnipeg, Man. (204) 983-7443; Calgary, Alta. (403) 292-5828; and New Westminister, B.C. (604) 666-8900.

Immunizing agents

There are two types of immunizing products: (1) vaccine, which contains inactivated virus and induces an active immune response beginning in 7 to 10 days and persisting for at least 1 year; (2) rabies immune globulin, human (RIG), which provides rapid protection that persists for only a short period of time (half-life about 21 days).

Vaccine and immune globulin should be used concurrently for optimum post-exposure prophylaxis against rabies, except in certain previously immunized persons, as indicated below. **Under no circumstances should vaccine be administered in the same syringe or at the same site as RIG.**

Table 1
Post-Exposure Prophylaxis for Persons Not Previously Immunized Against Rabies

Animal species	Condition of animal at time of exposure	Management of exposed person
Dog or cat	Healthy and available for 10 days' observation	1. Local treatment of wound 2. At first sign of rabies in animal, give RIG (local and intramuscular) and start HDCV
	Rabid or suspected rabid* Unknown or escaped	1. Local treatment of wound 2. RIG (local and intramuscular) and HDCV
Skunk, bat, fox, coyote, raccoon and other carnivores. Includes bat found in room when a person was sleeping unattended.	Regard as rabid unless geographic area is known to be rabies free*	1. Local treatment of wound 2. RIG (local and intramuscular) and HDCV
Livestock, rodents or lagomorphs (hares and rabbits)	Consider individually. Consult appropriate public health and Food Inspection Agency officials. Bites of squirrels, chipmunks, rats, mice, hamsters, gerbils, other rodents, rabbits and hares may rarely warrant post-exposure rabies prophylaxis if the behaviour of the biting animal was highly unusual	

RIG = (human) rabies immune globulin, HDCV = human diploid cell vaccine
* If possible, the animal should be humanely killed and the brain tested for rabies as soon as possible; holding for observation is not recommended. Discontinue vaccine if fluorescent antibody test of animal brain is negative.

Vaccine

Post-exposure prophylaxis should be started as soon as possible after exposure and should be offered to exposed persons regardless of the elapsed interval. When notification of an exposure is delayed, prophylaxis may be started as late as 6 or more months after exposure. Vaccine should be administered in conjunction with RIG and should be given intramuscularly into the deltoid muscle (never in the gluteal region) or the anterolateral upper thigh in infants.

Five doses of 1 mL of HDCV should be given, the first dose (on day 0) as soon as possible after exposure, and additional doses on each of days 3, 7, 14 and 28 after the first dose. An appropriate dose of RIG, as described below, should also be given on day 0. Other immunization schedules have also been validated by the WHO. Routine follow-up of antibody levels is not necessary.

The course of vaccine may be discontinued if the direct fluorescent antibody test of the brain of an animal killed at the time of attack proves to be negative.

Rabies immune globulin

A dose of 20 IU/kg of RIG should be administered once, as soon as possible after exposure. Up to one half the dose should be infiltrated around the wound, if practical; the remainder should be given intramuscularly into the gluteal area or lateral thigh muscle (because of the large volume to be injected). When more than one wound exists, each should be locally infiltrated with a portion of the RIG. Because of interference with active antibody production, the recommended dose should not be exceeded. Since vaccine-induced antibodies begin to appear within 1 week, there is no value in administering RIG more than 8 days after initiating a vaccine course.

Post-exposure prophylaxis of previously immunized persons

Post-exposure prophylaxis for persons who have previously received rabies vaccine differs depending on whether an immune (neutralizing antibody) response was demonstrated or was highly likely to have developed, as would be the case after completed courses of immunization with approved vaccines and schedules.

A. Two doses of HDCV, one injected immediately and the other 3 days later, without RIG, are recommended for exposed individuals with the following rabies immunization history:
   i) Completion of an approved course of pre- or post-exposure prophylaxis with HDCV;
   ii) Completion of immunization with other types of rabies vaccine or with HDCV according to unapproved schedules but in whom neutralizing rabies antibody is demonstrated in serum.

B. A complete course of HDCV plus RIG is recommended for persons who may have received rabies vaccines but do not fulfil the criteria listed in A. A serum sample may be collected before vaccine is given, and if antibody is demonstrated the course may be discontinued, provided at least two doses of HDCV have been administered.

Pre-Exposure Vaccination

Pre-exposure rabies vaccination is an elective procedure and should be offered to persons at potentially high risk of contact with rabid animals, e.g., certain laboratory workers, veterinarians, animal control and wildlife workers, spelunkers and certain travellers (see page 194).

Three doses of HDCV are required, one on days 0, 7 and 21. The vaccine should be given as a 1.0 mL dose intramuscularly into the deltoid muscle. Post-vaccination rabies antibody determinations are not normally required but may be advisable for those anticipating frequent exposure or whose immune response may be reduced by illness, medication or advanced age. There is no licensed preparation for intradermal use in Canada.

Booster doses of vaccine

Persons with continuing high risk of exposure, such as certain veterinarians, should have their serum tested for rabies antibodies every 2 years; others working with live rabies virus in laboratories or vaccine-production facilities who are at risk of inapparent exposure should be tested every 6 months. Those with inadequate titres should be given a booster dose of HDCV. Persons previously immunized with other vaccines should be given sufficient doses of HDCV to produce an adequate antibody response.

Delayed systemic allergic reactions (see Adverse Reactions) appear to be less likely following booster doses of the vaccine purified by zonal centrifugation (Rabies Vaccine Inactivated [Diploid Cell origin]-Dried). This vaccine is therefore recommended for persons requiring ongoing protection against rabies.

An acceptable antibody response is considered to be a titre of 1:32 by the rapid fluorescent-focus inhibition test.

Adverse Reactions

HDCV: Local reactions such as pain, erythema, swelling and itching at the injection site may occur in 30% to 74% of recipients; mild systemic reactions such as headache, nausea, abdominal pain, muscle aches and dizziness may occur in about 20%. Systemic allergic reactions characterized by generalized urticaria and accompanied in some cases by arthralgia, angioedema, fever, nausea and vomiting have been reported. These reactions are uncommon in persons receiving primary vaccination but have occurred in up to 7% of persons receiving a booster dose, with onset after 2 to 21 days. These reactions have been shown to follow the development of IgE antibodies to beta propiolactone-altered human serum albumin in the vaccine. Vaccines purified by zonal centrifugation appear less likely to be associated with such reactions. Immediate anaphylactic reactions have occurred in 1 in 10,000 persons given HDCV. Neurologic complications are rare, but three cases of neurologic illness resembling Guillain-Barré syndrome, which resolved without sequelae within 12 weeks, have been reported.

RIG: Local pain and low grade fever may follow administration of RIG.

Precautions and Contraindications

A history of any previous hypersensitivity reaction to HDCV should be elicited. Hypersensitive individuals should be vaccinated only under strict medical supervision.

There is no contraindication to the use of rabies vaccine after significant exposure to a proven rabid animal.

Serious allergic or neuroparalytic reactions occurring during the administration of rabies vaccine pose a serious dilemma. The risk of rabies developing must be carefully considered before a decision is made to discontinue vaccination. The use of corticosteroids as a possible treatment may inhibit the immune response. The patient's blood should be tested for rabies antibodies and expert opinion should be sought in the management of these individuals.

Corticosteroids and immunosuppressive agents may interfere with the development of active immunity. Therefore, persons receiving steroids or immunosuppressive therapy should have a rabies antibody determination upon completion of a post-exposure course of rabies vaccine to ensure that an adequate response has developed.

Pregnancy is not a contraindication to post-exposure prophylaxis, but it would be prudent to delay pre-exposure vaccination of pregnant women unless there is a substantial risk of exposure.

SELECTED REFERENCES

Baer GM, Fishbein DB. *Rabies post-exposure prophylaxis.* N Engl J Med 1987;316:1270-72.

CDC. *Rabies prevention — United States, 1991: recommendations of the Immuniz-ation Practices Advisory Committee (ACIP).* MMWR 1991;(RR-3):1-19.

Dietzschold B, Ertl HCJ. *New developments in the pre- and post-exposure treatment of rabies.* Crit Rev Immunol 1991;10:427-39.

Fishbein DB, Dressen DW, Holmes DF et al. *Human diploid cell rabies vaccine purified by zonal centrifugation: a controlled study of antibody response and side effects following primary and booster preexposure immunizations.* Vaccine 1989;7:437-42.

Rupprecht CE, Smith JS, Fekadu M et al. *The ascension of wildlife rabies: a cause for public health concern or intervention?* Emerg Infect Dis 1995;1:107-13.

Varughese PV, Carter AO. *Rabies and post-exposure rabies prophylaxis in Canada, 1987-1988.* CDWR 1990;16:131-36.

Rabies Vaccine

RUBELLA VACCINE

Rubella is a viral disease of childhood, which may be difficult to diagnose clinically. Up to 50% of infections are subclinical. About 2,000 cases are reported annually in Canada.

Between October 1996 and June 1997, an outbreak of rubella occurred in Manitoba, involving over 3,600 cases. Approximately 90% of cases were males, with the highest attack rate in those 15-19 years. Most were unvaccinated. In Manitoba, a selective vaccination policy targeting prepubertal girls was practised for a number of years. Consequently, some male cohorts are susceptible. An MMR immunization program for all infants was introduced in April 1983 throughout Canada.

The major objective of vaccination is the prevention of rubella infection in pregnancy in order to prevent congenital rubella syndrome (CRS). This syndrome can result in miscarriage, stillbirth and fetal malformations, including congenital heart disease, cataracts, deafness and mental retardation, which may not become manifest for several years. The risk of fetal damage after maternal infection is particularly high in the earliest months after conception (85% in the first trimester) with progressive diminution of risk thereafter, and is very uncommon after the 20th week of pregnancy. Infected infants who appear normal at birth may later show eye, ear or brain damage. Congenital infection may become chronic and give rise to such problems as diabetes mellitus and panencephalitis later in life. An average of three cases of CRS have been reported annually in recent years.

Preparations Used for Immunization

Rubella virus vaccine currently licensed in Canada contains a live attenuated virus, strain RA 27/3, prepared in human diploid cell culture. The vaccine is administered as a subcutaneous injection and is available as a monovalent vaccine or in combination with mumps and measles vaccines (MMR) or measles vaccine (MR). It stimulates the formation of antibodies to rubella virus in over 97% of susceptible individuals. Titres are generally lower than those observed in response to natural rubella infection.

Antibody levels developed in response to earlier rubella vaccines decline over time, but this decline may not have great significance, since any detectable concentration of antibody generally protects against viremic infection. The duration of protection is not yet known, but studies indicate that it exceeds 20 years. Booster doses are not considered necessary but are not harmful and may provide a marginal benefit in protecting the population. Vaccine protection, based on available data, is expected to be lifelong. A documented history of vaccination is presumptive evidence of immunity.

Rubella Vaccine

Small quantities of vaccine strain virus may be detected in the nasopharynx of some vaccinees 7 to 28 days after vaccination, but transmission to contacts has not been conclusively documented. Therefore, it is safe to administer vaccine to persons in contact with susceptible pregnant women or immunocompromised persons.

Asymptomatic reinfection, manifested by a rise in antibody levels, has been observed in vaccinees and in women with naturally acquired immunity and very low antibody titres. Rarely, viremia may occur, and it is possible for a woman immune by natural disease or prior immunization to be reinfected while pregnant, but even more rare for her to transmit the virus to her fetus.

Recommended Usage
Infants and children
Two doses of live rubella vaccine are recommended routinely for all children, the first dose given on or as soon as practicable after their first birthday in combination with measles and mumps vaccines, and the second dose given at least 1 month later in combination with measles vaccine. Rubella vaccine should not be administered before 12 months of age. Although the rationale for administering two doses of measles-rubella containing vaccines is largely to provide optimal protection against measles, a second dose of rubella vaccine is not harmful and may provide a marginally increased level of protection in the population. Rubella-containing vaccines may be administered at the same time but at a separate injection site as DPT-containing vaccines routinely given at 18 months and school entry. Immunization schedules and requirements vary by province and territory, and can be obtained from the local public health department. A clinical history of rubella is not a reliable indicator of immunity.

Adolescents and adults
Rubella vaccine should be given to all female adolescents and women of childbearing age unless they have proof of immunity, as demonstrated by documented evidence of having received vaccine, or laboratory evidence of detectable antibody. At the first visit, rubella immunization status should be assessed. If there is no documentation of prior rubella immunization, one dose of rubella vaccine should be given using a measles-rubella containing vaccine, as a high proportion of rubella unvaccinated women may also be susceptible to measles. Routine serologic testing is not recommended as there are no known adverse effects specific to the administration of vaccine to immune women, and serologic testing may delay needed immunization.

Canadian, U.K. and Australian studies indicate that immigrant women from countries where rubella vaccine is not routinely used (e.g., the majority of Asian, African and many Caribbean and South and Central American countries) are at particular risk of being susceptible to rubella. Every effort should be made to immunize such adolescents and women as soon as possible or, for women who are pregnant on presentation, immediately post-partum.

In educational institutions, such as schools, colleges and universities, particular emphasis should be placed on immunization of susceptible female staff and female students of childbearing age because of their relatively high risk of exposure.

In health care settings, the rubella immunity status of female employees of childbearing age should be carefully reviewed, and those without documented immunity should be vaccinated. In addition, vaccine should be given to susceptible persons of either sex who may, through frequent face-to-face contact, expose pregnant women to rubella.

Serologic testing for rubella antibody should be a routine procedure during prenatal care for those without written serologic evidence of immunity or prior immunization. Since up to one third of cases of CRS occur in second and subsequent pregnancies, it is essential that all women found to be susceptible during pregnancy should receive rubella vaccine (preferably given as MMR vaccine) in the immediate post-partum period. Every effort should be made to immunize prior to hospital discharge. Canadian, U.S. and U.K. studies show that a large proportion of rubella-susceptible women are not immunized post-partum.

Anti-Rho(D) immune globulin may interfere with response to rubella vaccine. Rubella-susceptible women who receive anti-Rho(D) immune globulin post-partum should either be given rubella vaccine at the same time and tested 3 months later for rubella immunity, or should be immunized with rubella vaccine 3 months post-partum, with follow-up ensured.

Breast-feeding is not a contraindication to rubella vaccination. Although vaccine virus has been detected in breast milk and transmission can occur, no illness has been reported in the infants.

Vaccine must not be administered less than 2 weeks before an immune globulin injection. When immune globulin has been administered, rubella vaccination should be delayed for 3 months; it should be delayed for 5 months if given as MMR vaccine (see Table 7, page 26). It has been shown that previous or simultaneous blood transfusion does not generally interfere with the antibody response to rubella vaccination. In such cases, however, it is recommended that a serologic test be done 6 to 8 weeks after vaccination to test the individual's immune status. If it is seronegative, a second dose of vaccine should be administered.

Laboratory tests for seroconversion after vaccination are unnecessary except in special situations as above. If a serologic test is done for some other reason and found to be negative despite a history of rubella vaccination, a repeat dose of vaccine may be given once. It is not necessary to repeat vaccination more than once even if subsequent serologic tests are also negative, because such individuals usually have other evidence of rubella immunity.

Rubella Vaccine

Passive Immunization

The use of immune globulin (IG) for post-exposure prophylaxis of rubella in susceptible women exposed in early pregnancy is not generally recommended. Infants with CRS have been born to women given IG soon after exposure, and there are no reliable data to indicate the effectiveness of this approach. This intervention should be considered only for pregnant women who have been exposed to rubella and are not considering termination of the pregnancy.

Adverse Reactions

Rash and lymphadenopathy occur occasionally. Transient arthritis or arthralgia may occur 7 to 21 days after vaccination. This is uncommon in children, but frequency and severity increase with age in susceptible post-pubertal females. Paresthesia or pain in the extremities lasting 1 week to 3 months has been reported rarely. However, the frequency and severity of adverse reactions are less than occur after natural disease. Serious adverse reactions are rare.

Contraindications

Inquiry regarding pregnancy should be made before vaccination. Administration of the vaccine to pregnant women should be avoided. Women of childbearing age should be advised to avoid pregnancy for 1 month after vaccination.

Rubella vaccine is occasionally administered to women who are subsequently found to have been pregnant at the time or who become pregnant after vaccination. Reassurance can be given that no fetal damage was observed in the babies of over 700 susceptible women who received vaccine during their pregnancies and carried them to term. The theoretical risk of teratogenicity, if any, is very small. Therefore, rubella vaccination of a woman who is pregnant or who becomes pregnant within 1 month should not be a reason to consider termination of pregnancy.

In common with other live vaccines, rubella vaccine should not be administered to patients whose immune mechanism is impaired as a result of disease, injury or therapy. Rubella immunization is recommended for HIV-infected children. Use of the vaccine has not been associated with serious adverse reactions, although the immune response may be impaired.

Rubella vaccine should not be administered to persons known to be hypersensitive to vaccine components, such as antibiotics, used in its preparation; this includes anaphylactic hypersensitivity to neomycin. Persons with egg hypersensitivity may be immunized with MMR vaccine (refer to page 7).

Management of Outbreaks

During outbreaks, persons at risk who have not been vaccinated or do not have serologic proof of immunity should be given vaccine promptly without prior serologic testing. A history of rubella illness is not a reliable indicator of immunity.

Even though rubella immunization has not been shown to be protective when given after exposure, it is not harmful. It will protect the individual in future if the current exposure does not result in infection.

Surveillance

Laboratory confirmation of suspected cases of rubella and CRS must be sought. All suspected and confirmed cases of rubella and CRS must be reported to the appropriate local or provincial/territorial public health authority.

Since rubella presents with a clinical spectrum that can be imitated by other common viral infections, the specific diagnosis, which is particularly important during outbreaks or during contacts between suspected cases and pregnant women, can be confirmed only by serodiagnostic laboratory methods or culture. A significant rising antibody titre between acute and convalescent post-illness serum samples is confirmatory, with the first sample taken within the first 7 days after illness and the second 10 days after the first. A more rapid confirmation may be obtained by demonstrating rubella-specific IgM antibody in a serum sample taken between 3 days and 1 month after rash onset. False-negative results may be obtained if the serum sample is taken too early or too late after the clinical illness.

Congenital infection may be confirmed by isolation of the virus in neonatal urine or nasopharyngeal secretions, detection of IgM antibody to rubella virus in blood or the persistence of antibody to rubella virus beyond the age of 3 months. Consultation with the regional public health laboratory will indicate the availability and applicability of various serodiagnostic procedures for rubella.

Rubella Vaccine

SELECTED REFERENCES

American College of Obstetricians and Gynecologists. *Rubella and pregnancy.* Int J Gynecol Obstet 1993;42:60-6.

Berkeley MIKB, Moffat MAJ, Russell D. *Surveillance of antibody to rubella virus in Grampian: closing the immunity gap.* BMJ 1991;303:1174-76.

Briss PA, Fehrs LJ, Hutcheson RH, Schaffner W. *Rubella among the Amish: resurgent disease in a highly susceptible community.* Pediatr Infect Dis J 1992;11:955-59.

CDC. *Rubella and congenital rubella syndrome — United States, January 1, 1991-May 7, 1994.* MMWR 1994;43:391-401.

Chernesky MA, Wyman L, Mahony JB et al. *Clinical evaluation of the sensitivity and specificity of a commercially available enzyme immunoassay for detection of rubella virus-specific immunoglobulin M.* J Clin Microbiol 1984:400-04.

Enders G, Nickerl-Pacher U, Miller E, Cradock-Watson JE. *Outcome of confirmed periconceptional maternal rubella.* Lancet 1988;I:1445-46.

Howson CP, Fineberg HV. *Adverse events following pertussis and rubella vaccines. Summary of a report of the Institute of Medicine.* JAMA 1992;267:392-96.

Lee SH, Ewert DP, Frederick PD, Mascola L. *Resurgence of congenital rubella syndrome in the 1990s. Report on missed opportunities and failed prevention policies among women of childbearing age.* JAMA 1992;267:16-20.

Miller CL. *Rubella in the developing world.* Epidemiol Infect 1991;107:63-8.

Miller E. *Rubella in the United Kingdom.* Epidemiol Infect 1991;107:31-42.

Miller E, Waight PA, Vurdien JE et al. *Rubella surveillance to December 1992: second joint report from the PHLS and National Congenital Rubella Surveillance Programme.* CDR Rev 1993;3:R35-40.

Peltola H, Heinonen OP, Valle M et al. *The elimination of indigenous measles, mumps, and rubella from Finland by a 12-year, two-dose vaccination program.* N Engl J Med 1994;331:1397-1402.

Robinson J, Lemay M, Vaudry WL. *Congenital rubella after anticipated maternal immunity: two cases and a review of the literature.* Pediatr Infect Dis J 1994;13:812-15.

Rubella Vaccine

SMALLPOX VACCINE

A Historical Note

Smallpox vaccination is no longer necessary. As a result of concerted global immunization and disease surveillance efforts, the World Health Organization published the Declaration of the Global Eradication of Smallpox in May 1980. Smallpox vaccination programs were terminated shortly afterwards. Eradication of this dreaded disease was one of the most significant advances in public health of the 20th century.

TETANUS TOXOID

Tetanus is an acute and often fatal disease caused by an extremely potent neurotoxin produced by *Clostridium tetani*. The organism is ubiquitous and its occurrence in nature cannot be controlled. Immunization is highly effective, provides long-lasting protection and is recommended for the whole population. Only two to seven cases of tetanus are now reported annually in Canada. No deaths have been recorded since 1991 (Figure 1).

Figure 1: Tetanus - Number of Cases and Deaths 1924-1997

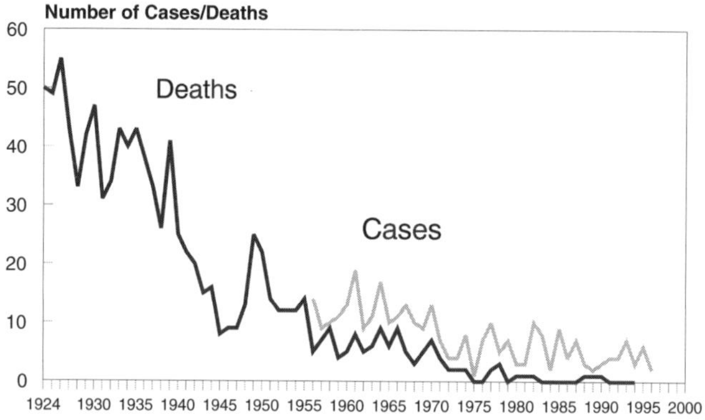

Tetanus toxoid introduced in 1940

Preparations Used for Immunization

Tetanus toxoid is prepared by detoxification of tetanus toxin with formalin. The toxoid is available in the plain (unadsorbed) form or combined with aluminum salts, generally aluminum phosphate, in the adsorbed form. Adsorbed toxoid is the agent of choice for primary immunization, but both forms are acceptable for booster doses.

The toxoid is available alone or in various combinations with diphtheria toxoid, pertussis vaccine and inactivated poliomyelitis vaccine. All preparations contain comparable amounts of tetanus toxoid.

Recommended Usage

Although tetanus toxoid may be used alone, adsorbed multiple-antigen vaccines are preferred for primary immunization because of the broader protection imparted. For children < 7 years of age, tetanus toxoid is most commonly used in combination with diphtheria toxoid and pertussis vaccine (DPT; or DT where a contraindication exists to pertussis). For persons ≥ 7 years of age, use of an adult-type preparation of tetanus and diphtheria toxoids (Td, adsorbed or Td-Polio) is recommended.

The primary immunizing course of tetanus toxoid (adsorbed), either alone or in combination with other antigens, consists of three doses, except in children < 7 years to whom a fourth dose is given. These children should also receive a booster dose at 4 to 6 years of age (school entry) if the fourth primary dose was given before the fourth birthday. In adults, the first two doses of toxoid (preferably as Td) should be given 4 to 8 weeks apart and the third 6 to 12 months later.

Active immunization of all Canadians against tetanus should be undertaken, even for patients who have recovered from this disease, because infection does not confer protective immunity. Tetanus toxoid preparations can be given concurrently with other vaccines in circumstances in which this would be advantageous.

To maintain immunity to tetanus following completion of primary immunization, booster doses administered as Td are recommended at 10-yearly intervals. More frequent boosters may lead to severe local and systemic reactions. Less frequent boosters may also suffice, as tetanus rarely develops in adults who have completed primary immunization but have not observed the recommendation for 10-yearly boosters. However, there are few firm data on which to base a recommendation for less frequent boosters, and it is known that antitoxin levels decline with time. At a minimum, children should receive the booster doses recommended at 4 to 6 and 14 to 16 years. Subsequently, immunization status should be reviewed at least once during adult life, e.g., at 50 years of age, and a dose of Td given to everyone who has not had one within the previous 10 years. (See also pages 54, 56 and 74-5.)

Booster immunization should also be considered in the event of tetanus-prone wounds (see next section). About 7% to 10% of tetanus cases occur without a recognized wound or burn beforehand.

Tetanus Prophylaxis in Wound Management

The following table summarizes the recommended use of immunizing agents in wound management. It is important to ascertain the number of doses of toxoid previously given and the interval since the last dose. The serum level of antitoxin considered to be protective is 0.01 International Units/mL. When a tetanus booster dose is required, the combined preparation of tetanus and diphtheria toxoid formulated for adults (Td) is preferred. Appropriate cleansing and debridement of wounds is imperative, and use of antibiotics may be considered.

Tetanus Toxoid

When travel to a developing country is planned more than 5 years after the last tetanus booster, it may be prudent to offer an early booster, since in some developing countries health care facilities may not be able to guarantee the safe administration of a booster dose if required.

Table 1
Guide to Tetanus Prophylaxis in Wound Management
(Check footnotes carefully.)

History of tetanus immunization	Clean, minor wounds		All other wounds	
	Td*	TIG†	Td	TIG
Uncertain or primary** immunization incomplete	Yes	No	Yes	Yes
Primary** immunization complete	Yes‡	No	Yes§	No¶

* Adult type tetanus and diphtheria toxoid. If the patient is < 7 years old, DT, DPT, DPT-polio, DPT-Hib, or DPT-Polio/Hib is given as part of the routine childhood immunization.
** Primary immunization is described in the text (Recommended Usage).
† Tetanus immune globulin.
‡ Yes, unless there is documentaion of a booster within the last 10 years.
§ Yes, unless there is documentation of a booster within the last 5 years. The bivalent toxoid, Td, is not considered to be significantly more reactogenic than T alone and is recommended for use in this circumstance. The patient should be informed that Td has been given.
¶ No, unless individuals are known to have a significant immune deficiency state (e.g., HIV, agammaglobulinemia) since immune response to tetanus toxoid may be suboptimal.

Adverse Reactions

Adverse reactions to primary immunization with tetanus toxoid are rare, especially in children. The incidence in adults increases with age. Following booster doses, local erythema and swelling are not uncommon but only occasionally severe. Severe local reactions are often associated with high levels of circulating antitoxin, usually as a result of over-immunization. Systemic reactions, such as generalized urticaria, are uncommon. Anaphylaxis and peripheral neuropathy have rarely been reported.

Contraindications and Precautions

It is recommended that tetanus toxoid not be given routinely to a patient who has received a booster dose in the preceding 5 years.

Tetanus toxoid should not be given if a severe systemic reaction followed a previous dose.

Persons who experience a major local reaction or high fever following a dose of tetanus toxoid should not be given another dose for at least 10 years. In those who have experienced severe local reactions or fever after tetanus toxoid, plain toxoid may be considered for subsequent booster doses, since it is reported to cause fewer reactions than adsorbed toxoid. When a contraindication to tetanus toxoid exists and a patient sustains a major or unclean wound, tetanus immune globulin should be given.

Before giving a combined vaccine, it is most important to ensure that there are no contraindications to the administration of any of the components.

There is no evidence that tetanus toxoid is teratogenic, but it is prudent to wait until the second trimester of pregnancy to administer a routinely required dose, to minimize any theoretic risk. In the event of a tetanus-prone wound during pregnancy the recommendations in the table should be followed. Neonatal tetanus may occur in infants born to unimmunized mothers under unhygienic conditions.

SELECTED REFERENCES

CDC. *Tetanus surveillance — United States, 1989-1990*. In: *CDC surveillance summaries*. MMWR 1992;41(No. SS-8):1-19.

LaForce M. *Routine tetanus immunizations for adults: once is enough*. J Gen Intern Med 1993;8:459-60.

Simonsen O, Badsberg JH, Kjeldsen K et al. *The fall-off in serum concentration of tetanus antitoxin after primary and booster vaccination*. Acta Pathol Microbiol Immunol Scand [C] 1986;94:77-82.

Simonsen O, Block AV, Klerke A et al. *Immunity against tetanus and response to revaccination in surgical patients more than 50 years of age*. Surg Gynecol Obstet 1987;164:329-34.

Simonsen O, Kjeldsen K, Heron I. *Immunity against tetanus and effect of revaccination 25-30 years after primary vaccination*. Lancet 1984;2:1240-42.

Simonsen O, Klaerke M, Jensen JEB et al. *Revaccination against tetanus 17 to 20 years after primary vaccination: kinetics of antibody response*. J Trauma 1987;27:1358-61.

Tetanus Toxoid

TYPHOID VACCINE

Typhoid fever is caused by *Salmonella typhi*, which differs from most other *Salmonella* species in that it infects only humans and frequently causes severe systemic illness. The organism is generally transmitted via food contaminated with the feces or urine of persons with the disease or those who are *S. typhi* carriers. The fatality rate is approximately 16% for untreated cases and 1% for those given appropriate antibiotic therapy. Between 2% and 5% of typhoid cases become chronic carriers, sometimes remaining so for years. The risk of severe illness is increased in persons with depressed immunity or decreased gastric acid levels.

In endemic areas (such as Africa, Asia, Central and South America), typhoid fever is primarily a disease of persons 5 to 19 years of age; cases in children < 5 years of age account for fewer than 5% of the total number, and typhoid fever in children < 2 years of age is infrequently reported. The reason for the lower risk of typhoid fever in children < 5 years of age is unclear, but the observation is important in light of our incomplete knowledge of vaccine immunogenicity and efficacy in this age group.

The incidence of typhoid fever is very low in all of the industrialized countries. Approximately 90 cases are reported in Canada annually. The low incidence of typhoid is attributable to improved living conditions, better quality of drinking water, and the treatment of sewage. The vaccine does not seem to play an important role in maintaining this lower incidence.

For travellers to areas where sanitation is likely to be poor, immunization is **not** a substitute for careful selection and handling of food and water, since the vaccine will not prevent disease in those who ingest a large number of organisms. However, vaccination is expected to further reduce the risk of typhoid fever among healthy visitors to areas with endemic disease.

Preparations Used for Immunization
Two typhoid vaccines are currently available for protection against typhoid fever.

Typhim Vi™ capsular polysaccharide vaccine
This vaccine is an injectable solution of Vi (virulence) antigen prepared from the capsular polysaccharide (ViCPS) of *S. typhi* strain TY2. The vaccine is produced by Pasteur Mérieux Connaught and distributed in Canada under the name of Typhim Vi™. Each 0.5 mL dose of vaccine contains 25 µg of polysaccharide, which stimulates a specific, humoral antibody response that confers protection against infection (i.e., at least a fourfold rise in antibody titre) in 93% of healthy adults. Controlled trials have demonstrated that the serologic response to vaccine correlated with protective efficacy.

Two randomized, double-blind, controlled field trials of ViCPS in disease-endemic areas demonstrated protective efficacy rates of 50% and 74%. The efficacy of vaccination with ViCPS has not been studied among persons from areas without endemic disease who travel to disease-endemic regions or among children < 5 years of age. ViCPS has not been tested among children < 1 year of age.

Oral live-attenuated Ty21a vaccine

Oral, live attenuated typhoid vaccine is supplied as liquid or enteric-coated capsules containing lyophilized Ty21a, a mutant strain of *S. typhi*. The vaccine stimulates a cell-mediated immune response as well as inducing both secretory and humoral antibody. Because vaccinees do not shed viable organisms in their stool, secondary transmission does not occur. Protective efficacy of 42% to 67% has been reported for the capsule formulation of the vaccine available in Canada. Oral live Ty21a vaccine prevented disease in 17% and 19% of school children 5 to 9 years of age in two different studies; in two others, protection rates were 54% and 72% among school children 10 to 19 years of age. Protection has persisted for up to 7 years. There are no data on the rate or duration of protection by oral typhoid vaccine for travellers from developed countries or for children < 5 years of age. Neither are there reports regarding the protective efficacy of the oral vaccine in persons previously vaccinated with parenteral vaccines.

Recommended Usage

Routine typhoid vaccination is not recommended in Canada. Selective vaccination should, however, be considered in the following groups:

1. Travellers who will have prolonged (> 4 weeks) exposure to potentially contaminated food and water, especially those travelling to or working in small cities, villages or rural areas in countries with a high incidence of disease. Vaccination is not routinely recommended for short-term (< 4 weeks) travel to resort hotels in such countries.

2. Persons with ongoing household or intimate exposure to an *S. typhi* carrier.

3. Laboratory workers who frequently handle cultures of *S. typhi*.

Typhoid vaccination is not recommended for workers in sewage plants, for controlling common-source outbreaks, for persons attending rural summer or work camps or for persons in nonendemic areas experiencing natural disasters such as floods. Typhoid vaccine is not recommended for the control or containment of typhoid outbreaks in Canada.

Typhoid vaccine does not confer complete protection against disease, and immunity may be overwhelmed by large inoculum of *S. typhi*. Therefore, it is advisable that vaccinees be warned that immunization is only one preventive measure against typhoid fever in an endemic country or high-risk situation, **and that care in selection of food and water is of primary importance.** They should also be reminded of the need for booster doses if they continue to be at risk.

Oral typhoid vaccine (Ty21a)

For adults and children ≥ 6 years of age, one enteric-coated capsule should be taken on alternate days to a total of four capsules. Each capsule should be taken on an empty stomach with a liquid no warmer than 37° C. The capsules must be kept refrigerated until they are used, and all four capsules must be taken for full protection. After storage for 7 days at 20-25° C, all lots evaluated met potency requirements.

A liquid preparation has been licensed recently that is reported to be more effective than the capsules. This liquid preparation (Vivotif Berna L Vaccine) is indicated for immunization of adults and children ≥ 3 years of age against diseases caused by *Salmonella typhi*. The recommendations in the package insert should be followed. It is essential that all three doses of vaccine be taken at the prescribed alternate day interval to obtain a maximal protective immune response. A recent study in Thailand demonstrated seroconversion rates of 83% after three doses of liquid vaccine in 4- to 6-year-old school children and reported no adverse reactions to immunization.

Antibiotics with activity against *S. typhi* or other Salmonellae may interfere with replication of the vaccine. Persons receiving therapy with such antibiotics should have vaccination deferred until at least 48 hours after completing the antibiotic course. Antimalarial prophylaxis, specifically mefloquine, may also interfere with vaccine replication. At least 8 hours should separate the administration of oral vaccine and a dose of mefloquine.

Since there are no data on safety or efficacy in young children, the manufacturer recommends oral typhoid vaccine not be given to children < 6 years of age.

Minor variations in dosing schedule are not expected to affect the efficacy of typhoid vaccination. However, if it is deemed necessary to repeat the series because of long intervals (> 4 days) between doses, the administration of an additional full course of vaccine would not be harmful.

Protection persists for at least 5 years after immunization. At the present time it is recommended to repeat the four doses of the oral vaccine every 7 years if the risk of disease exposure persists.

No experience has been reported using oral typhoid vaccine as a booster for persons previously vaccinated with the parenteral vaccine. However, using a series of four doses of oral vaccine is a reasonable alternative to a parenteral booster dose.

Since the vaccine is self administered, compliance issues must be considered in its selection.

Parenteral, Vi capsular polysaccharide vaccine

For adults and children ≥ 2 years of age, a single dose of 0.5 mL (25 µg) given intramuscularly is recommended.

The optimum interval for booster doses has not been established, but the manufacturer recommends booster doses every 3 years if continued or renewed exposure is expected. The duration of vaccine-induced protection is not well established. In follow-up studies the ViCPS vaccine maintained its protective efficacy at 17 months and 21 months; however, Vi antibody has been observed to decline by about 35% at 11 months and by about 60% at 27 months after immunization.

There are no data on the use of this vaccine as a booster for persons who have received a primary series with another vaccine. However, a single dose of the vaccine at the appropriate interval should re-establish protection.

Adverse Reactions

Several lots of the oral typhoid vaccine have been evaluated in field trials both in adults and in school-aged children. Objectively monitored side effects, e.g., abdominal pain, diarrhea, vomiting, fever, headache and skin rash, did not occur at a statistically higher frequency in the vaccinated group than in the placebo group.

The parenteral Vi capsular polysaccharide vaccine produces reactions only half as frequently as the previous inactivated vaccine. Fever (4% to 10%), headache (7% to 27%) and erythema and induration at the injection site (4% to 18%) have been reported.

Contraindications and Precautions

Oral live typhoid vaccine is contraindicated in anyone with hypersensitivity to any component of the vaccine or the enteric-coated capsule. It should not be given to immunocompromised or immunosuppressed persons, including those with known HIV infection; neither should it be given during an acute febrile illness or to any person with acute gastrointestinal disease or chronic inflammatory bowel disease.

Oral typhoid vaccine should not be given to pregnant women.

Safe storage should be emphasized in households with small children.

The administration of oral typhoid and oral cholera vaccine should be separated by at least 8 hours.

For parenteral ViCPS, the only contraindication is a history of a severe local or systemic reaction to a previous dose of this vaccine. Although this highly purified vaccine would not be expected to have any adverse effects, its safety in pregnancy has not been directly studied. Therefore, the benefits of vaccine must be carefully weighed against any potential adverse effects before it is given to pregnant women.

SELECTED REFERENCES

Acharya IL, Lowe CU, Thapa R et al. *Prevention of typhoid fever in Nepal with the Vi capsular polysaccharide of Salmonella typhi.* N Engl J Med 1987;317:1101-04.

Barnett ED, Chen R. *Children and international travel: immunizations.* Pediatr Infect Dis J 1995;14:988-89.

CDC. *Typhoid immunization recommendations of the Advisory Committee on Immunization Practices (ACIP).* MMWR 1994;43:RR-14.

Committee to Advise on Tropical Medicine and Travel (CATMAT). *Statement on overseas travelers and typhoid.* CCDR 1994;20:61-2.

Cryz SJ Jr. *Post-marketing experience with live oral Ty21a vaccine.* Lancet 1993;341:49-50.

Horowitz H, Carbonaro CA. *Inhibition of the Salmonella typhi oral vaccine strain, TY21a, by mefloquine and chloroquine.* J Infect Dis 1992;166:1462-64.

Ivanoff B, Levine MM, Lambert PH. *Vaccination against typhoid fever: present status.* Bull WHO 1994;72:957-71.

Keitel WA, Bond NL, Zahradnik JMB et al. *Clinical and serological responses following primary and booster immunization with Salmonella typhi Vi capsular polysaccharide vaccines.* Vaccine 1994;12:155-59.

Klugman KP, Gilbertson IT, Koornhof HJ et al. *Protective activity of Vi capsular polysaccharide vaccine against typhoid fever.* Lancet 1987;2:1165-69.

Levine MM, Ferrecio C, Black RE et al. *Comparison of enteric coated capsules and liquid formulation of Ty21a typhoid vaccine in randomized controlled field trial.* Lancet 1990;2:891-94.

Levine MM, Ferrecio C, Black RE et al. *Large scale field trial of Ty21a live oral typhoid vaccine in enteric-coated capsule formulation.* Lancet 1987;1:1049-52.

Levine MM, Taylor DN, Ferrecio C. *Typhoid vaccine come of age.* Pediatr Infect Dis J 1989;8:374-81.

Mahle WT, Levine MM. *Salmonella typhi infection in children younger than 5 years of age.* Pediatr Infect Dis J 1993;12:627-31.

YELLOW FEVER VACCINE

Yellow fever is endemic in the tropical areas of Africa and Central and South America, but has never been seen in Asia. The disease may occur in two epidemiologic forms — urban, and sylvatic or jungle. Both forms are caused by the same virus. Urban outbreaks occur as a result of transmission by the mosquito *Aedes aegypti*, which is widely distributed throughout the tropics. Jungle yellow fever is a disease of monkeys in the forests of Central and South America and Africa, which is transmitted by forest mosquitoes to humans, e.g., to forestry or oil company employees. A recent resurgence of yellow fever in certain countries prompted WHO to include yellow fever vaccine routinely within the Expanded Programme on Immunization.

Disease control includes protection from mosquitoes, elimination of *A. aegypti* from urban areas, and immunization of forest workers and urban residents who are at risk of exposure. Unimmunized Canadians can acquire yellow fever when travelling abroad but cannot transmit the disease on their return to Canada, since the recognized mosquito vectors do not occur in this country.

Preparations Used for Immunization

Yellow fever vaccine is a live vaccine prepared in chick embryos from the attenuated 17D strain. The lyophilized preparation should be stored at the temperature specified by the manufacturer until it is reconstituted by the addition of the recommended diluent. Unused vaccine must be discarded 1 hour after reconstitution. The vaccine has proved to be extremely safe and effective.

Recommended Usage

The vaccine is recommended for all travellers passing through or living in countries in Africa, Central America and South America where yellow fever infection is officially reported. It is also recommended for travel outside the urban areas of countries that do not officially report yellow fever but lie in the yellow fever "endemic zones" (see Maps 1 and 2).

Vaccination is required by law upon entry to certain countries irrespective of the traveller's country of origin, and in other countries when travellers are coming from endemic areas. In some cases, vaccination against yellow fever is recommended, even though not required by law, e.g., if yellow fever has been reported in the country of destination. In some Asian and other tropical countries where yellow fever does not exist but the transmitting mosquito is present, vaccination is required for arrivals from an endemic country to prevent importation of the disease. Current information on the countries for which an International Certificate of Vaccination is required can be obtained from local health departments.

Map 1
Yellow Fever Endemic Zones in Africa

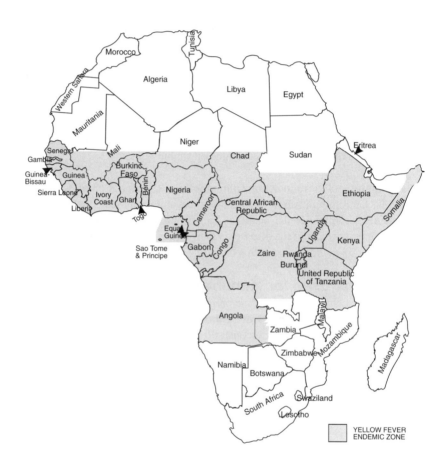

Source: WHO. *International travel and health: vaccination requirements and health advice.*
            Geneva: WHO, 1997.

Map 2
Yellow Fever Endemic Zones in the Americas

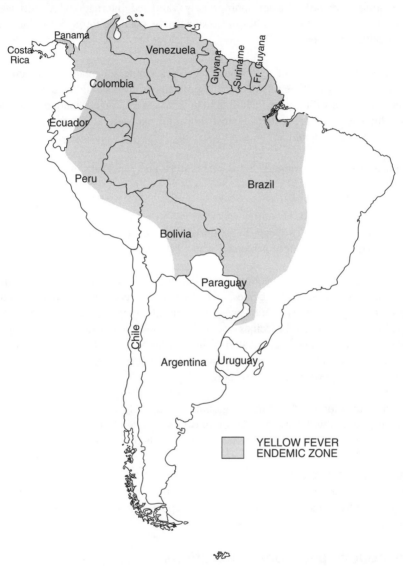

YELLOW FEVER
ENDEMIC ZONE

Source: WHO. *International travel and health: vaccination requirements and health advice.* Geneva: WHO, 1997.

Yellow Fever Vaccine

For purposes of international travel, yellow fever vaccine is administered only at a Yellow Fever Vaccination Centre approved by Health Canada and the WHO, and the vaccination is recorded in an appropriately validated International Certificate of Vaccination. A list of such centres in Canada can be obtained through provincial and local health departments.

Travellers ≥ 9 months of age should receive a single subcutaneous injection of vaccine. Infants 4 to 9 months of age and pregnant women should be considered for immunization only if they are travelling to high-risk areas, travel cannot be postponed and a high level of prevention against mosquito exposure is not feasible. Infants < 4 months of age should not be given vaccine.

Vaccination is also recommended for laboratory personnel who work with yellow fever virus.

Immunity develops 10 days after vaccination and persists for more than 10 years. Revaccination every 10 years is required for travel to endemic areas and is recommended for laboratory personnel who work with the virus.

The serologic response to yellow fever vaccine is not inhibited by concurrent administration of other live vaccines, including live oral cholera and live oral typhoid vaccines. If live vaccines are not given concurrently, they should be spaced at least 4 weeks apart. Inactivated vaccines, except inactivated cholera vaccine, may be given concurrently or at any interval after yellow fever vaccine. Inactivated parenteral cholera vaccine and yellow fever vaccine should be given 3 or more weeks apart to avoid interference with antibody responses.

The administration of immune globulin and yellow fever vaccine either simultaneously or within a short span of time does not alter the immunologic response, because immune globulin is unlikely to contain antibody to yellow fever virus.

Adverse Reactions

About 5% of vaccinees have mild headache, myalgia, low grade fever or other minor symptoms 5 to 10 days after vaccination. Encephalitis has occurred rarely in young infants.

Precautions and Contraindications

Infants < 4 months of age should not be vaccinated because of the risk of encephalitis after vaccination, which may occur in as many as 1% of infants < 3 months of age. Vaccination of children 4 to 9 months old and pregnant women should be avoided unless they are likely to be exposed to an ongoing epidemic of yellow fever. Yellow fever vaccine should not be given to persons whose immune mechanisms are suppressed by disease or therapy. HIV-infected individuals should not be vaccinated unless they will be at actual risk of exposure to yellow fever, as already defined.

Because yellow fever vaccine is prepared from chick embryos, it should not be given to individuals with known anaphylactic hypersensitivity to the ingestion of eggs, manifested as hives, swelling of the mouth and throat, difficult breathing, hypotension and shock. If vaccination of an individual with a questionable history of egg hypersentivity is considered essential because of a high risk of exposure, an intradermal test dose may be administered under close medical supervision. Specific directions for skin testing are found in the package insert.

SELECTED REFERENCES

Barnett ED, Chen R. *Children and international travel: immunizations*. Pediatr Infect Dis J 1995;14:982-92.

Coursaget P, Fritzell B, Blondeau C et al. *Simultaneous injection of plasma derived or recombinant hepatitis B vaccines with yellow fever and killed polio vaccines*. Vaccine 1995;13:109-11.

Döller C. *Vaccination of adults against travel-related infections, diseases, and new developments in vaccines*. Infection 1993;21:7-23.

Kollavitsch H, Que JU, Wiedermann X et al. *Safety and immunogenicity of live oral cholera and typhoid vaccines administered alone or in combination with antimalaria drugs, oral polio vaccine and yellow fever vaccine*. J Infect Dis 1997;175:871-75.

Tsai TF, Paul R, Lynberg MC et al. *Congenital yellow fever virus infection after immunisation in pregnancy*. J Infect Dis 1993;163:1520-23.

WHO. *International travel and health: vaccination requirements and health advice*. Geneva: WHO, 1997.

Part 4
PASSIVE IMMUNIZING AGENTS

Protection against certain infections or a reduction in the severity of the illness they cause can be achieved by administration of preformed antibodies derived from humans or animals. The preparations available are of two types: standard immune globulin (IG) of human origin, sometimes referred to as "immune serum globulin" or "gamma globulin"; and special preparations of either human or animal sera containing high titres of specific antibodies to a particular microorganism or its toxin, such as tetanus immune globulin. Products of human origin are preferred over those of animal origin because of the high incidence of adverse reactions to animal sera and the longer lasting protection conferred by human globulins.

Passive immunization should be considered when vaccines for active immunization are not available or are contraindicated, or in certain instances when vaccines have not been used before exposure to the infective agent, as may be the case when an unimmunized patient sustains a wound that may be contaminated with tetanus bacilli. In the latter situation, passive immunization is used in combination with toxoid to ensure both immediate (conferred by passive immunization) and long-term protection. Passive immunization may also have a role in the management of immunosuppressed persons unable to respond to a vaccine. The beneficial effects provided by passive immunizing agents are of relatively short duration, and protection may be incomplete.

In these guidelines, emphasis is on the prophylactic use of immune sera, and only brief reference is made to their use as therapeutic agents in established infections.

As with all immunizing agents, including these blood-derived products, the risks and benefits need to be explained before administration, and the lot number should be recorded.

Immune Globulin (Human)

Immune globulin (IG) is a sterile, concentrated solution containing between 100 g/L and 180 g/L (10% to 18%) of protein and the preservative thimerosal. It is obtained from pooled human plasma and contains mainly IgG with small amounts of IgA and IgM. The potency of each lot of final product of immune globulin is tested against international standards or reference preparations for at least two different antibodies, one viral and one bacterial. IG is stable for prolonged periods when stored at $2°$ to $8°$ C. Maximum plasma levels are reached about 2 days after intramuscular injection, and the half-life in the recipient's circulation is 21 to 27 days.

Intravenous immune globulin (IGIV) is a preparation that contains 50 g/L (5%) protein with maltose, sucrose or glycine as a stabilizing agent. It is used for continuous passive immunization in patients with selected congenital or acquired immunoglobulin deficiency states and certain diseases. Detailed discussion of IGIV is beyond the scope of this document. Consult appropriate sources and the manufacturer's package instructions.

Recommended Usage

Prophylactic use of IG has been shown to be effective in a limited number of clinical situations. Commonly recommended doses are used in the following situations; however, the dose may vary by manufacturer, and recommendations in the package inserts should be followed.

1. Measles

IG can be given to prevent or modify measles in susceptible persons within 6 days after exposure. To prevent disease, it should be given as soon as possible after exposure, preferably within 3 days. The recommended dose is 0.25 mL/kg of body weight with a maximum dose of 15 mL. The dose of IG for exposed individuals who have underlying malignant disease or who are otherwise immunologically deficient is 0.5 mL/kg or 15 mL maximum.

IG should be considered for susceptible contacts of measles, particularly all children < 1 year of age, and immunologically compromised individuals for whom measles vaccine is contraindicated. Susceptible immunocompetent individuals who present within 4 to 6 days after exposure, i.e., too late for vaccine, can also be considered for IG. When clinical measles does not develop in a person given IG, measles vaccine should be given 5 months later, provided the individual is ≥ 1 year of age and there are no contraindications to the vaccine.

IG should not be used in an attempt to control measles outbreaks.

2. Hepatitis A

Hepatitis A vaccine is the preferred method of pre-exposure prophylaxis against hepatitis A. IG may be indicated for post-exposure prophylaxis, as detailed in the chapter Hepatitis A Vaccine (see pages 87-88).

3. Rubella

IG given soon after exposure to rubella may modify or suppress symptoms but is not certain to prevent infection, including congenital infection. Therefore, the routine use of IG in susceptible women early in pregnancy who are exposed to rubella is not recommended, although it may be considered when termination of pregnancy is not acceptable. A dose of 0.55 mL/kg may be given intramuscularly within 48 hours of

Part 4 – Passive Immunizing Agents

contact. Serum rubella antibody measurements before and for several months after IG administration can determine whether infection occurred.

4. Hepatitis C

IG is not efficacious in preventing or treating hepatitis C and should not be used.

Safety of IG Preparations

Human IG preparations are among the safest blood-derived products available. Plasma found positive for hepatitis B surface antigen, HIV antibody or hepatitis C is excluded from donor pools. The method of preparation includes one or more steps that exclude or inactivate hepatitis B and C, and HIV. There are no known reports of transmission of hepatitis B, hepatitis C, HIV or other infectious agents after the intramuscular injection of IG. There have been rare reports of transmission of hepatitis B or hepatitis C following use of certain intravenous IG preparations that did not undergo the currently required inactivation steps during the manufacturing process. None of these products was ever commercially available in Canada.

Adverse Reactions

Reactions at the site of injection include tenderness, erythema and stiffness of local muscles, which may persist for several hours. Mild fever or malaise may occasionally occur. Less common side effects include flushing, headache, chills and nausea. Anaphylactic reactions may occur rarely with repeat administration.

Contraindications

IG should not be given to persons with known isolated IgA deficiency or with a known allergy to the preservative thimerosal, a mercury derivative. Pregnancy is not a contraindication to the use of IG or other immune globulins.

Precautions

Currently available preparations, with the exception of IGIV, must not be given intravenously because of the risk of rare anaphylactic reactions.

Large volumes for intramuscular injection should be divided and injected at two or more sites.

Persons with severe thrombocytopenia or coagulation disorders that contraindicate intramuscular injections should not be given intramuscular IG unless the expected benefits outweigh the risks.

IG administration may interfere transiently with the subsequent immune response to measles, mumps and rubella vaccines. See Table 7, page 26 for specific recom-mendations regarding the recommended interval between the administration of IG and these vaccines.

There are no data to indicate that immune globulin administration interferes with the response to inactivated vaccines, toxoids or the following live vaccines: yellow fever or the oral preparations of typhoid, cholera or polio.

Specific Immune Globulins

Specific immune globulins are derived from the pooled sera of persons with antibody to the specific infectious agents. Antisera from animals, usually horses that are hyper-immunized against a specific organism, are used when human products are not available. Because of the relatively high risk of serum sickness following the use of animal products, human immune globulin should be used whenever possible. *Before antisera of animal origin is injected, testing for hypersensitivity to the preparation should be carried out in accordance with the manufacturer's recommendation.*

1. Botulism antitoxin (equine)

Trivalent (type A, B and E) and monovalent (type E) antitoxin preparations, both containing phenol as a preservative, are available on an emergency basis (consult with local public health authorities). These products are used prophylactically in persons suspected of having eaten food contaminated with botulism toxin, and therapeutically in persons with established or suspected botulism. Type E botulism is most likely to be associated with the consumption of uncooked fish or fish products or the flesh of marine mammals, including whales and seals. The monovalent type E antitoxin should be used only if such foodstuffs are considered the most likely vehicle of disease or if laboratory tests have established that the toxin involved is type E. In populations at risk for repeated exposures to botulism toxin because of particular food habits, the repeated use of prophylactic antitoxin can lead to an increased incidence of severe reactions. Caution should therefore be exercised in the use of botulism antitoxin in such circumstances, even if preliminary sensitivity tests are negative.

2. Diphtheria antitoxin (equine)

This preparation, which also contains phenol as a preservative, is available on an emergency basis (consult with local public health authorities) for treatment of the disease. Antitoxin should be administered before bacteriologic confirmation when there is clinical suspicion of diphtheria. The method for testing for sensitivity to equine serum as well as the dose and route of administration are indicated in the manufacturer's package insert. Intramuscular administration usually suffices, but intravenous administration may be necessary in some cases. If sensitivity tests are positive, desensitization must be undertaken according to the manufacturer's recommendations.

Diphtheria antitoxin is not recommended for prophylaxis in close, unimmunized contacts of diphtheria cases, given the substantial risk of allergic reaction to horse serum and no evidence of additional benefit of antitoxin for contacts who have received antimicrobial prophylaxis.

3. Hepatitis B immune globulin (HBIG)

HBIG is prepared from pooled human plasma from selected donors with a high level of antibody to hepatitis B surface antigen. The indications for use are percutaneous or mucosal exposure to blood containing hepatitis B virus, sexual contact with an acute case of hepatitis B, and birth of an infant to a mother with acute or chronic hepatitis B infection (see pages 96-99 for details of use).

4. Rabies immune globulin (RIG)

Passive immunization with this product is undertaken as part of post-exposure prophylaxis against rabies (see pages 153-154).

5. Respiratory syncytial virus immune globulin intravenous (human) (RSV-IGIV)

RSV-IGIV is an intravenous IG derived from pools of human plasma with high concentrations of protective antibodies that neutralize RSV. RSV-IGIV was approved in August 1997 for prevention of RSV infection among children aged < 2 years old with bronchopulmonary dysplasia (BPD) or a history of premature birth (≤ 35 weeks' gestation). Rates of readmission for RSV infection among premature infants have ranged from 2% to 22% during the first year of life and require further study. RSV-IGIV in a placebo-controlled trial was shown to decrease the RSV-related hospitalization rate by 41%, the RSV-related length of stay by 53% and the duration of oxygen therapy by 60%.

Adverse events are as for all IG products given by intravenous infusion. Fluid overload may be precipitated by infusion to infants with pulmonary disease, especially those with BPD. Appropriate precautions, as outlined in the product monograph, must be taken.

Children with cyanotic congenital heart disease treated with RSV-IGIV were observed to have a greater frequency of severe or life-threatening adverse events than similar children who received no infusions during the study period. Until the relationship between the infusions and subsequent adverse events is better understood it is recommended that children with cyanotic congenital heart disease not be given RSV-IGIV. It is unknown whether RSV-IGIV can prevent significant RSV disease among immunocompromised hosts.

RSV-IGIV has no proven benefit in the treatment of established RSV infection.

It is anticipated that RSV-IGIV prophylaxis may be most beneficial for the following children:

- Infants and children < 2 years with BPD who are currently receiving or have received oxygen therapy within 6 months before the start of the RSV season.

- Infants who were born at 32 weeks of gestation or less, including those without BPD:

  - infants born at 28 weeks of gestation or less may benefit from prophylaxis up to 12 months of age;

  - infants born at 29-32 weeks of gestation may benefit from prophylaxis up to 6 months of age.

Local and practical issues in delivery, costs, and the data showing that prevention is *not* complete after administration of RSV-IGIV all preclude a universal recommendation being made at this time. Thus each centre has to consider a number of factors before embarking upon an RSV-IGIV prophylaxis program. The use of RSV-IGIV may not prove to be very feasible or practical in many centres when these factors or circumstances are taken into account.

The recommended dose is 750 mg/kg given every 4 weeks starting before and continuing through the local RSV season. In Canada, the annual RSV outbreak usually begins in November or December and extends through April or May. Regional variations occur. It is best to consult local experts to determine the usefulness of RSV-IGIV on an individual patient basis. A more detailed discussion can be found in the statement published by the Canadian Paediatric Society as referenced below.

6. Tetanus immune globulin (TIG)

The use of TIG in the management of wounds is discussed in the section on Tetanus Toxoid (see pages 165-166). When used in the treatment of tetanus, TIG should be administered intramuscularly in an effort to neutralize tetanus toxin in body fluids. It has no effect on toxin already fixed to nerve tissue. The optimal therapeutic dose has not been established.

7. Varicella-zoster immune globulin (VZIG)

VZIG is prepared from pooled plasma of persons with high antibody titres to varicella-zoster virus (VZV). VZIG is available through Canadian Red Cross distribution centres.

Passive immunization with VZIG is indicated after exposure to chickenpox or zoster in susceptible individuals whose risk of serious morbidity or mortality from chickenpox is substantially increased.

Persons with chickenpox are most contagious from 1 to 2 days before and for a few days after onset of the rash. The contagious period may extend to 5 days after onset and in immunocompromised patients until crusting of lesions. Skin lesions of zoster

Part 4 – Passive Immunizing Agents

183

or shingles are infectious only until the eruption has crusted and dried. The following contact situations are considered significant exposures to VZV:

- continuous household contact (living in the same dwelling)

- playing indoors for more than 1 hour with a contagious case

- sharing the same hospital room with a contagious patient

- prolonged face-to-face contact of a worker or staff member with an individual with chickenpox.

The determinants of susceptibility to varicella are as follows:

- Persons with a history of chickenpox are usually considered immune.

- All recipients of heterologous bone marrow transplants should be considered susceptible in the early post-transplantation period regardless of a past history of varicella or positive serology.

- Persons with a negative or uncertain history of chickenpox should be tested serologically to establish susceptibility, since as many as 70% to 95% of such individuals have immunity to varicella. Prospective serologic testing to determine susceptibility may eliminate the need for emergency post-exposure tests. Prospective testing should be considered for health care workers without a history of chickenpox, and for individuals with congenital or acquired immunodeficiency due to disease or therapy, including those undergoing solid-organ heterograft transplantation, and those with hematologic or reticuloendothelial malignant disease. VZIG may give detectable levels of antibody causing false-positive tests of varicella immunity for up to 2 months after administration.

VZIG is recommended for the following susceptible persons, providing significant exposure has occurred:

a) *Infants and children*
   1. Immunocompromised patients, such as those with congenital or acquired immunodeficiency due to disease or treatment, including some patients receiving corticosteroid therapy (see pages 18-19). Patients receiving regular monthly infusions of 100 to 400 mg/kg of IGIV and whose most recent dose was within 3 weeks before exposure do not require VZIG.
   2. Newborn infants of mothers who develop varicella during the 5 days before or 48 hours after delivery.
   3. Hospitalized premature infants exposed during the first weeks of life. Exposed infants of < 28 weeks' gestational age should receive VZIG regardless of maternal immune status. Exposed infants of 29 to 37 weeks' gestational age should receive VZIG if the mother was not immune.

b) *Adults*

    1. Pregnant women. Because the risk of complications of chickenpox in pregnant women may be greater than in other adults, VZIG should be given to exposed, susceptible pregnant women. There is no evidence that VZIG will prevent or alter disease in the fetus.

    2. Immunocompromised adults. See previous section on immunocompromised infants and children and page 16.

    3. Normal adults. The value of VZIG in normal adults is unclear. Chickenpox can be more severe in normal adults than children, but the risk of pneumonia is now considered less than was formerly believed. In addition, VZIG may prolong the incubation period to 28 days, which has implications for health care workers. Finally, acyclovir therapy initiated within 24 hours after onset of the rash is effective in accelerating skin lesion healing and is thus a therapeutic alternative to prophylactic VZIG.

The recommended dose of VZIG is 125 units (1 vial) per 10 kg body weight to a maximum of 625 units, administered intramuscularly. The optimal dose for adults is uncertain.

VZIG is of benefit if administered within 96 hours after the exposure. Protection is believed to last for 3 to 4 weeks. Subsequent exposures more than 3 weeks after a dose of VZIG may require additional doses.

Part 4 – Passive Immunizing Agents

SELECTED REFERENCES

Buckley RH, Schiff RI. *The use of intravenous immune globulin in immunodeficiency diseases.* N Engl J Med 1991;325:110-17.

Canadian Paediatric Society Committee on Immunization and Infectious Diseases. *Respiratory syncytial virus – immune globulin intravenous (RSV-IVIG).* Paediatr Child Health 1998;3:11-4.

Gershon AA. *Chickenpox, measles and mumps.* In: Remington JS, Klein JO, eds. *Infectious diseases of the fetus and newborn infant.* 3rd ed. Philadelphia: WB Saunders, 1990:395-445.

McIntosh D, Isaacs D. *Varicella zoster virus infection in pregnancy.* Arch Dis Child 1993;68:1-2.

Miller E, Cradock-Watson JE, Ridehalgh MKS. *Outcome in newborn babies given anti-varicella-zoster immunoglobulin after perinatal maternal infection with varicella-zoster virus.* Lancet 1989;2:371-73.

Patou G, Midgley P, Meurisse EV et al. *Immunoglobulin prophylaxis for infants exposed to varicella in a neonatal unit.* J Infection 1990;20:207-13.

The PREVENT Study Group. *Reduction of respiratory syncytial virus hospitalization among premature infants and infants with bronchopulmonary dysplasia using respiratory syncytial virus immune globulin prophylaxis.* Pediatrics 1997;99:93-9.

Siber GR, Snyderman DR. *Use of immune globulins in the prevention and treatment of infections.* In: Remington JS, Swartz MN, eds. *Current clinical topics in infectious diseases.* Vol. 12. Boston: Blackwell Scientific,1992:208-56.

Siber GR, Werner BC, Halsey NA et al. *Interference of immune globulin with measles and rubella immunization.* J Pediatr 1993;122,2:204-11.

Part 5
IMMUNIZATION OF HEALTH CARE WORKERS AND OTHERS PROVIDING PERSONAL CARE

Hospital employees, students in health care disciplines, laboratory workers and other health care personnel are at risk of exposure to communicable diseases because of their contact with patients or material from patients with infections, both diagnosed and undiagnosed. Maintenance of immunity against vaccine-preventable diseases is an integral part of a health care facility's occupational health program. Optimal usage of immunizing agents in hospital staff will not only safeguard the health of staff members but may, in some instances, also protect patients from becoming infected by hospital employees. In certain circumstances, family members should also be considered as health care workers, since they provide a significant and growing amount of care and because in-home transmission of infectious disease is recognized.

The immunization status of each worker should be assessed at the time of initial employment. A full vaccination history should be elicited and efforts made to obtain documentation of the doses received and dates of administration. Persons who cannot provide acceptable information or evidence of adequate immunity should be offered immunization at the earliest opportunity. Records of all immunizations and serologic tests should be kept by both employer and employee and a recall system for boosters instituted.

Immunization policies at individual institutions will vary, and decisions about which vaccines to be included should take account of the size and nature of the institution, the exposure risks for the health care worker and the nature of employment. It is important to include increased acceptance of vaccinations as an educational objective in employee in-service as well as increased awareness of illnesses or symptoms that require evaluation.

Vaccines Recommended for All Health Care Workers

Diphtheria and tetanus toxoid
Immunization against diphtheria and tetanus is recommended for all adults in Canada. The opportunity should be taken on entry into health care employment to ensure that the appropriate series and booster doses have been given. Booster doses of Td are recommended every 10 years for optimal protection.

Measles vaccine

Newly employed health care workers born after 1970 who have patient contact should have proof of two live measles vaccinations, documentation of physician-diagnosed measles or laboratory evidence of immunity. For health care workers who have already received one dose of measles vaccine, a second dose of vaccine is recommended generally as MMR vaccine. Persons born before 1970 have probably been infected naturally and may usually be considered immune. It is not necessary to initiate a serologic testing program to detect susceptible health care workers.

Polio vaccine

Primary immunization with inactivated poliomyelitis vaccine (IPV) is indicated for all health care workers who may be exposed to poliovirus and have not had a primary course of poliovirus vaccine (OPV or IPV). OPV is not recommended for health care workers because they may shed the virus and inadvertently expose immunocompromised patients to live virus. Persons who have not been given a full primary course should have the series completed with IPV regardless of the interval since the last dose. Booster doses of IPV are not required for health care workers in Canada.

Rubella vaccine

In health care settings, the rubella immune status of female employees of childbearing age should be carefully reviewed, and those without documented immunity should be vaccinated with MMR unless there are contraindications. In addition, vaccine should be given to susceptible persons of either sex who may, through frequent face-to-face contact, expose pregnant women to rubella. Women should be advised to avoid pregnancy for 1 month after vaccination.

Hepatitis B vaccine

Hepatitis B vaccine is recommended for health care workers and others who may be exposed to blood or blood products, or who may be at increased risk of sharps injury, bites or penetrating injuries (for example, clients and staff of institutions for the developmentally challenged). Health care workers who have been exposed either percutaneously or through the mucous membranes to a source that is known or is likely to be positive for hepatitis B surface antigen should be assessed for the need for hepatitis B vaccine and immune globulin according to the recommendations outlined in the chapter on hepatitis B (see pages 97-98).

Influenza vaccine

Annual influenza vaccination is recommended for all health care personnel who have contact with individuals in high-risk groups. Such personnel include physicians, nurses and others in both hospital and outpatient settings; employees of chronic care facilities who have contact with residents; and providers of home care, visiting nurses or volunteers, and household members of persons at high risk. Influenza vaccination of health care workers has been shown to reduce the mortality and morbidity of patients under their care in long-term settings and to reduce worker illness during the influenza season.

Acetaminophen (650 mg taken 4, 8 and 12 hours after vaccination) has been shown to significantly reduce the incidence of side effects such as sore arm and nausea, and may reassure those for whom concern about side effects is an impediment to vaccination. Vaccination should be available in the workplace.

Other vaccines

Indications for the use of other licensed vaccines are generally the same for health care workers as for the general population. However, some vaccines may also be indicated for certain workers believed to be at particularly high risk of exposure, such as laboratory workers in specialized reference or research facilities. For example, typhoid vaccination should be considered for laboratory staff who frequently handle cultures of *S. typhi*.

Specific Risk Situations
Hepatitis A

Prevention of hepatitis A transmission within a hospital should be based on the use of good hygienic practices and patient care techniques, especially proper hand washing and management of potentially infected materials.

There may be other limited indications for hepatitis A vaccine.

For those who are not immune and who have had unusually close contact with patients with hepatitis A, such as direct oral exposure to patients' secretions or excretions soon after the onset of illness, immune globulin should be given.

BCG vaccine

Comprehensive application of infection control practices remains the primary strategy to protect health care workers from infection with *M. tuberculosis*. However, outbreaks of multidrug-resistant tuberculosis in health care settings have led to a reconsideration of BCG vaccination for health care workers in some situations. BCG vaccination may be considered for health care workers (including medical laboratory workers) at considerable risk of exposure to tubercle bacilli, especially drug-resistant bacilli, in situations in which protective measures against infection are known to be ineffective or not feasible.

SELECTED REFERENCES

Advisory Committee on Immunization Practices (ACIP) and the Hospital Infection Control Practices Advisory Committee. *Immunization of health-care workers.* Atlanta, Georgia: US Department of Health and Human Services, Public Health Service, Centers for Disease Control and Prevention. October 8, 1996.

Aoki FY, Yassi A, Cheang M, Math M et al. *Effects of acetaminophen on adverse effects of influenza vaccination in health care workers.* Can Med Assoc J 1993;149:1425-30.

Brewer TF, Colditz GA. *BCG vaccination for the prevention of tuberculosis in health care workers.* Clin Infect Dis 1995; 20:136-42.

Clever LH, LeGuyader Y. *Infectious risks for health care workers.* Annu Rev Public Health 1995;16:141-64.

Diekema DJ, Doebbeling BN. *Employee health and infection control.* Infect Control Hosp Epidemiol 1995;16:192-301.

Doebbeling BN, Ning Li MB, Wenzel RP. *An outbreak of hepatitis A among health care workers: risk factors for transmission.* Am J Public Health 1993;83:1679-84.

Furesz J, Scheifele DW, Palkonyay L. *Safety and effectiveness of the new activated hepatitis A virus vaccine.* Can Med Assoc J 1995;152:343-48.

Gardner P, Schaffner W. *Immunization of adults.* N Engl J Med 1993;328:1252-58.

Krause PJ, Gross PA, Barrett TL et al. *Quality standards for assurance of measles immunity among health care workers.* Infect Control Hosp Epidemiol 1994;15:193-99.

Murata PJ, Young LC. *Physicians' attitudes and behaviors regarding hepatitis B immunization.* J Fam Pract 1993;36:163-68.

Oakley K, Gooch C, Cockcroft A. *Review of management of incidents involving exposure to blood in a London teaching hospital, 1989-91.* BMJ 1992;304:949-51.

Potter J, Stott DJ, Roberts MA, Elder AG, O'Donnell B, Knight PV, Carman WF. *Influenza vaccination of health care workers in long-term care hospitals reduces the mortality of elderly patients.* J Infect Dis 1997;175:1-6.

Schwarz S, McCaw B, Fukushima P. *Prevalence of measles susceptibility in hospital staff: evidence to support expanding the recommendations of the Immunization Practices Advisory Committee.* Arch Intern Med 1992;152:1481-83.

Part 6
IMMUNIZATION OF TRAVELLERS

A detailed discussion of immunization and other preventive measures required for travellers to other countries is beyond the scope of this guide. Readers are referred to *Health Information for International Travel* (U.S. Centers for Disease Control and Prevention); *International Travel and Health: Vaccination Requirements and Health Advice* (WHO); the LCDC FAXlink service (dial 613 941-3900); and Health Canada's home page on the World Wide Web (http://www.hc-sc.gc.ca).

The immunization recommendations for travel will vary according to the traveller's age, existing medical conditions, the nature of travel (whether the traveller is staying in urban hotels or visiting remote rural areas), the legal requirements for entry into countries being visited and the duration of travel. Current information on vaccination requirements and recommendations should be obtained from public health agencies or travel health clinics.

There is no single schedule for the administration of immunizing agents to travellers. Each schedule must be personalized according to the individual traveller's immunization history, the countries to be visited, the type and duration of travel, and the amount of time before departure.

With some notable exceptions, most immunizing agents can be given simultaneously at different sites. Concerns about individual vaccines and their potential compatibility with other vaccines or antimicrobials (including antimalarials) are dealt with in the specific vaccine chapters of this guide.

A health care provider or travel medicine clinic should be consulted 2 to 3 months in advance of travel in order to allow sufficient time for optimal vaccination schedules to be completed.

It must be emphasized that the most frequent health problems faced by international travellers are not preventable by immunizing agents. As well, immunization is not a substitute for careful selection and handling of food and water.

Keeping the above considerations in mind, health care providers should consider the following immunizations for travellers.

Vaccinations Required as a Condition of Entry

1. Yellow fever

Yellow fever vaccination is the only one required as a condition of entry under the World Health Organization's International Health Regulations. A valid International Certificate of Vaccination, issued within the past 10 years, is mandatory for entry into certain countries in Africa and South America. Other countries have requirements for proof of vaccination from travellers who have passed through a yellow fever zone (see maps on pages 174-175). The period of validity of the International Vaccination Certificate for yellow fever is 10 years, beginning 10 days after primary vaccination and immediately after revaccination. The decision to vaccinate against yellow fever will depend on the itinerary of the individual traveller and the specific requirements of the countries to be visited (including stopovers).

Only designated yellow fever vaccination clinics can provide the International Certificate of Vaccination in Canada. For more information on the clinics and international certificates please contact Quarantine and Migration Health, LCDC (phone 613-957-8739, fax 613-952-8286).

2. Other

Individual countries may require particular vaccination in special circumstances (e.g., meningococcal vaccine for pilgrims to Mecca during the Hajj).

Recommended Vaccinations

Tourists are generally at lower risk of infection than persons who intend to live and work in foreign countries. Nevertheless, all persons travelling overseas are advised to ensure that their own routine immunizations are up to date to avoid diseases such as diphtheria, which reappeared in epidemic form in countries of the former USSR in the early 1990s. Persons planning to travel off the usual tourist routes or work in another country may need to take special precautions, such as receiving typhoid vaccine and hepatitis B vaccines. In specific circumstances, cholera, rabies, meningococcal or Japanese encephalitis vaccines may be useful.

The use of these vaccines should be considered in consultation with a health care provider or in accordance with the recommendations of medical authorities in the countries to be visited.

1. Poliomyelitis

The risk of polio for travellers has substantially decreased as we move towards global eradication. Travellers who plan to visit an area where polio is endemic or epidemic should be adequately immunized. In general, travellers do not require any polio vaccination if they have been given a complete primary course of oral poliovirus vaccine (OPV) or inactivated poliovirus vaccine (IPV). In adults, if the polio immunization status is unclear, a single dose of IPV may be given if more than 10 years have elapsed since the last dose of vaccine. Further doses during adulthood are not required. For partially immunized or unimmunized persons, refer to the poliomyelitis section in this guide.

2. Measles
Two doses of measles vaccine are recommended for all unimmunized travellers aged ≥ 1 year who were born after 1970 and who are en route to a measles endemic area, unless there is serologic proof of immunity or physician documentation of prior measles.

3. Rubella
A single dose in combination with measles and mumps vaccine is recommended for all unimmunized children and for susceptible women of child-bearing age.

4. Tetanus and diphtheria
Boosters are recommended every 10 years for optimal protection. When travel to a developing country is planned more than 5 years after the last tetanus booster, it may be prudent to offer an early booster, since in some developing countries health care facilities may not be able to guarantee the safe administration of a booster dose if required.

5. Typhoid
Typhoid vaccine is recommended for travellers who will have prolonged exposure to potentially contaminated food and water, especially those travelling to smaller cities and villages or rural areas off the usual tourist itineraries. Currently, there is a parenteral and a live oral vaccine available.

There may be an interaction between the live oral vaccine and concurrently used antimicrobials (including antimalarials). Please refer to the typhoid chapter of the guide.

6. Hepatitis B
Travel is a good opportunity to offer hepatitis B immunization to those who have not been previously vaccinated. It should be recommended particularly to travellers residing in areas with high levels of endemic hepatitis B or working in health care facilities, and those who are likely to have contact with blood or sexual contact with residents of such areas.

7. Hepatitis A
Hepatitis A is the most common vaccine-preventable disease in travellers. Protection against hepatitis A is recommended for travellers to developing countries, especially to rural areas or areas where the hygienic quality of the food and water supply is likely to be poor and hepatitis A is endemic.

Active immunization with hepatitis A vaccine is the first choice for protection against hepatitis A for travellers. One dose of the vaccine provides prompt, effective protection and should be followed by a second dose 6 to 12 months after the first (as recommended for the specific product) for travellers needing long-term protection. The vaccine is available alone or in combination with hepatitis B vaccine.

Protective antibodies are detectable within 2 weeks of administration, and therefore there should not be a need to give concurrent immune globulin.

Passive immunization with immune globulin provides protection for only 3 to 5 months and should be given immediately before departure. It may be recommended in special circumstances (e.g., children under the age of 1 year).

8. Rabies

Pre-exposure immunization should be considered for persons intending to live or work in areas where rabies is enzootic and where rabies control programs for domestic animals are inadequate. If such pre-exposure immunization is given, administration of two booster doses is imperative as soon as possible after exposure to a rabid animal, since pre-exposure immunization may not provide adequate protection.

9. Meningococcal disease

One dose of a quadrivalent vaccine is recommended for travellers planning a prolonged stay in areas with a high incidence of meningococcal disease. Short-term travellers (< 3 weeks) staying in city hotels and having little contact with the local population are at minimal risk and do not need to be vaccinated. However, in special circumstances vaccination should be considered for short-term travellers if (a) there will be close contact with the local population in endemic areas, (b) there will be travel to epidemic areas or (c) the traveller will be providing health care to others.

Meningococcal vaccine may be required by certain countries, e.g., Saudi Arabia for pilgrims to Mecca during the Hajj.

10. Japanese encephalitis

Japanese encephalitis occurs throughout most of East Asia from India to Korea and Japan. It occurs in epidemics in late summer and early fall in temperate areas, including Korea, and sporadically throughout the year in tropical areas of Southeast Asia, including Thailand. The vaccine is recommended for travel of > 4 weeks in rural areas of endemic countries.

11. Cholera

In specific, limited circumstances, the oral live cholera vaccine may be considered for travellers. The parenteral, inactivated cholera vaccine offers limited effectiveness and is not recommended.

There may be interaction between the oral live cholera vaccine and concurrently used antimicrobials (including antimalarials). Please refer to the cholera chapter of the guide.

12. BCG

Vaccination with BCG may be considered for travellers planning extended stays in areas of high tuberculosis prevalence, particularly where a program of serial skin testing and appropriate chemoprophylaxis may not be feasible or where primary isoniazid resistance of *Mycobacterium tuberculosis* is high. Travellers are advised to consult a specialist in travel medicine or infectious diseases when considering a decision for or against BCG immunization. Please refer to the appropriate chapter in the guide.

13. Influenza

People at high risk of influenza complications embarking on foreign travel to destinations where influenza is likely to be circulating should be vaccinated with the most current available vaccine. In the tropics, influenza can occur throughout the year. In the southern hemisphere, peak activity occurs from April through September and in the northern hemisphere from November through March. Influenza transmission is enhanced in the crowded conditions associated with air travel, cruise ships and tour groups.

Travel Immunization for Infants and Young Children

Infants and children should be up to date on all routine immunizations for their age. Modifications to the routine immunization schedule and additional vaccines that may be recommended for travel are outlined below.

1. Diphtheria, pertussis, tetanus, polio and *Haemophilus influenzae* type b (Hib)

An accelerated series for both DPT-P and Hib can be offered prior to travel, with doses spaced 4 to 6 weeks apart. See the appropriate sections in the guide.

2. Measles

Measles vaccine should be given at an earlier age for children travelling to countries where measles is endemic. It may be given as monovalent measles vaccine as early as 6 months of age, but then the primary series of two doses must be restarted after the child is 12 months old.

3. Yellow fever

Immunization of infants carries an increased risk of encephalitis. Children < 4 months of age should not be vaccinated. Vaccination of children 4 to 9 months of age should be avoided unless they are travelling to an area epidemic for yellow fever. If vaccination is required for entry but the infant will not be at risk of infection, a medical waiver should be provided.

4. Hepatitis B

Travel is a good opportunity to offer immunization to infants and young children who have not been previously vaccinated. It should be recommended particularly if they will live in an area where hepatitis B is endemic.

5. Hepatitis A

The same criteria used to recommend protection against hepatitis A for an adult traveller should be used for children. For children < 1 year of age, immune globulin may be considered.

6. Typhoid

The same criteria used to recommend vaccination against typhoid for an adult traveller should be used for children. Oral typhoid vaccine (capsules) is not recommended under the age of 6 years. A liquid preparation has recently been licensed and can be used in children as young as 3 years. The parenteral vaccine is not recommended under the age of 2 years.

7. Meningococcal disease

If indicated because of travel to a risk area for group A disease, vaccine may be given to infants as young as 3 months. The efficacy of the vaccine against group C disease is less for children < 2 years of age. See pages 126-128 for details regarding number and timing of doses.

8. Cholera

The same criteria used to recommend vaccination against cholera for adults should be used for children. The oral cholera vaccine is not recommended under the age of 2 years.

9. Japanese encephalitis

The same criteria used to recommend vaccination against Japanese encephalitis for an adult traveller should be used for children. Vaccination is not recommended under the age of 1 year.

10. Rabies

Children living in areas where rabies is enzootic and who are too young to understand the need to avoid animals or to report traumatic contacts should be considered for pre-exposure vaccination, at the same dose as for adults.

11. BCG

Vaccination with BCG may be considered for travellers planning extended stays in areas of high tuberculosis prevalence, particularly where a program of serial skin testing and appropriate chemoprophylaxis may not be feasible or where primary isoniazid resistance of *Mycobacterium tuberculosis* is high. Travellers are advised to consult a specialist in travel medicine or infectious diseases when considering a decision for or against BCG immunization. Please refer to the appropriate chapter in the guide.

Malaria Prophylaxis

Travellers should be advised about the two important measures to prevent malaria infection: avoiding mosquito bites and using antimalaria medication. Current information concerning malaria, drug-resistant strains of *Plasmodium,* as well as recommended drugs for prophylaxis and other preventive measures is regularly updated by the Committee to Advise on Tropical Medicine and Travel (CATMAT) and published in the Canada Communicable Disease Report (CCDR). Information is also available from local health departments, travel clinics, or the Laboratory Centre for Disease Control, Health Canada (LCDC FAXlink service [dial 613-941-3900] and Health Canada's home page on the World Wide Web [http://www.hc-sc.gc.ca]).

Travellers Who are Immunodeficient or Infected with HIV

See the appropriate section of the guide for recommendations on the use of vaccines in immunodeficient persons.

SELECTED REFERENCES

CDC. *Health information for international travel 1996-1997.* Atlanta: DHHS, 1997.

WHO. *International travel and health: vaccination requirements and health advice.* Geneva: WHO, 1997.

APPENDIX I
DEFINITIONS USED FOR REPORTABLE
ADVERSE EVENTS

Consult the facsimile of the reporting form included in this Guide for definitions. The following notes are clarifications and amplifications, where necessary, of the definitions or notations on the reporting form.

Adenopathy
Report severe or unusual enlargement or drainage of the lymphatic nodes.

Allergic Reaction
Indicate whether therapy with antihistamines was found clinically necessary and/or useful.

Anaphylaxis
Should be distinguished from vaso-vagal episodes. If unsure whether it was true anaphylaxis (epinephrine given rapidly), describe the episode as completely as possible while noting the uncertainty. True anaphylaxis is rare.

Anesthesia/Paresthesia
Describe patient symptoms and course of illness in detail.

Arthralgia/Arthritis
Note any pre-existing history of arthritis, as well as any diagnostic testing done, and persistence of symptoms if follow-up information available.

Convulsion/Seizure
Episodes shortly after vaccination are more likely secondary to the act of vaccinating (i.e., features of a vaso-vagal episode). Note if this is the suspected etiology. Otherwise, carefully note the presence or absence of fever, as well as any antipyretic use.

Encephalopathy
Describe symptom onset and clinical course.

Fever
Report temperatures 39° C or above (rectal equivalent) or believed high with accompanying systemic symptoms.

Guillain-Barré Syndrome
Indicate if the patient had any other recent illnesses (GBS may have an antecedent viral etiology).

Hypotonic-Hyporesponsive Episode
This condition is non-specific. Follow definition carefully but report any possible cases. Tends to be related to pertussis-containing vaccines.

Infected Abscess
If antibiotics have been prescribed for a possible cellulitis, and signs and symptoms appear to have responded to the treatment, code this definition.

Meningitis and/or Encephalitis
Describe symptom onset and clinical course.

Paralysis
Differentiate from weakness or immobility due to pain (which may be seen in children).

Parotitis
Swelling and/or tenderness of the parotid glands.

Rashes
No need to code those that are part of an allergic reaction, but descriptions of all rashes should be made.

Screaming Episode/Persistent Crying
The key is the persistence and abnormal character (for that infant). Should be differentiated from a dramatic pain response if possible.

Severe Pain and/or Severe Swelling
Lasting for at least 4 days, or requires hospitalization.

Severe Vomiting and/or Diarrhea
Note the possibility of any co-existing illness that may be responsible.

Sterile Abscess/Nodule
Since small nodules are common, report those that are significant; usually this means that they persist for > 1 month and are > 2.5 cm in diameter.

Thrombocytopenia
Please indicate laboratory values and/or basis for the diagnosis.

Other Severe or Unusual Events

Describe any other reaction that is significant enough to warrant reporting. Please include reason for reporting (of medical/epidemiologic interest, dramatic, not listed in product information, unexpected, patient very concerned, etc.). Indicate a specific diagnosis in addition to clinical description.

APPENDIX II

■✦■ Health Canada   Santé Canada

REPORT OF A VACCINE-ASSOCIATED ADVERSE EVENT
Protected when completed

IDENTIFICATION

PATIENT IDENTIFIER	PROVINCE/TERRITORY	DATE OF BIRTH	YEAR	MONTH	DAY	SEX	DATE OF VACCINE ADMINISTRATION	YEAR	MONTH	DAY
						☐ Male ☐ Female				

VACCINES

VACCINE(S) GIVEN	NUMBER IN SERIES	SITE	ROUTE	DOSAGE	MANUFACTURER	LOT NUMBER

ADVERSE EVENT(S) *Events marked with an asterisk (*) must be diagnosed by a physician.* Report only events which cannot be attributed to co-existing conditions. Additional information for all events should be provided under SUPPLEMENTARY INFORMATION on reverse side. Record interval between vaccine administration and onset of each event in minutes, hours or days.

LOCAL REACTION AT INJECTION SITE

☐ INFECTED ABSCESS (tick one or both of the options below)   MIN. HOURS DAYS
 (i) positive gram stain or culture ☐
 (ii) existence of purulent discharge with inflammatory signs ☐

☐ STERILE ABSCESS/NODULE   MIN. HOURS DAYS
No evidence of acute microbiological infection

☐ SEVERE PAIN AND/OR SEVERE SWELLING   MIN. HOURS DAYS
(tick one or both of the options below)
 (i) lasting 4 days or more ☐
 (ii) extending past nearest joint(s) ☐

☐ SCREAMING EPISODE/PERSISTENT CRYING   MIN. HOURS DAYS
Inconsolable for 3 hours or more; OR quality of cry definitely abnormal for child and not previously heard by parents

☐ FEVER   MIN. HOURS DAYS
Highest recorded temperature (Report only 38.0°C (102.2° F) or above)
 Temperature: _____ °C (or _____ °F)
 Site: rectal ☐ oral ☐ axilla ☐ skin ☐ tympanic ☐
 Temperature believed to be high but not recorded ☐
 Should be supported by the presence of other systemic symptoms

☐ ADENOPATHY (tick one or both of the options below)   MIN. HOURS DAYS
 (i) enlarged lymph node(s) ☐
 (ii) drainage of lymph node(s) ☐
 Site(s) _____

☐ PAROTITIS   MIN. HOURS DAYS
Swelling with pain and/or tenderness of parotid gland(s)

*☐ ANAPHYLAXIS OR SEVERE SHOCK   MIN. HOURS DAYS
Explosive, occurring within minutes after immunization, and evolving rapidly towards cardiovascular collapse AND requiring resuscitative therapy

☐ OTHER ALLERGIC REACTIONS (tick one or more of the options below)   MIN. HOURS DAYS
 (i) wheezing or shortness of breath due to bronchospasm ☐
 (ii) swelling of mouth or throat ☐
 (iii) skin manifestations (e.g., hives, eczema, pruritus) ☐
 (iv) facial or generalized edema ☐

☐ RASHES (other than hives)   MIN. HOURS DAYS
Lasting 4 days or more AND/OR requiring hospitalization
 Generalized ☐ Localized (indicate site) ☐ _____
 Specify characteristics of rash _____

☐ ARTHRALGIA/ARTHRITIS   MIN. HOURS DAYS
Joint pain/inflammation lasting at least 24 hours
If condition is an acute exacerbation of a pre-existing diagnosis, give details under Supplementary Information

☐ SEVERE VOMITING AND/OR DIARRHEA   MIN. HOURS DAYS
Must be severe enough to interfere with daily routine

☐ HYPOTONIC-HYPORESPONSIVE EPISODE (in children < 2 yrs, only)   MIN. HOURS DAYS
Characterised by all the features of: (i) generalized decrease/loss of muscle tone; AND (ii) pallor or cyanosis; AND (iii) decreased level of awareness or loss of consciousness
Should not be mistaken for fainting, a post-convulsion state, or anaphylaxis

☐ CONVULSION/SEIZURE   MIN. HOURS DAYS
 Febrile ☐   Afebrile ☐
 Past history of: A) Febrile seizures Yes ☐ No ☐
                   B) Afebrile seizures Yes ☐ No ☐
Omit fainting, seizures occurring within 30 minutes of immunization, and seizures occurring as part of encephalopathy or meningitis/encephalitis

*☐ ENCEPHALOPATHY   MIN. HOURS DAYS
Acute onset of major neurological illness characterized by any two or more of: (i) seizures; (ii) distinct change in level of consciousness or mental status (behaviour and/or personality) lasting 24 hours or more; (iii) focal neurological signs which persist for more than 24 hours

*☐ MENINGITIS AND/OR ENCEPHALITIS   MIN. HOURS DAYS
Abnormal CSF findings AND an acute onset of: (i) fever with neck stiffness or positive meningeal signs; OR (ii) signs and symptoms of encephalopathy (see ENCEPHALOPATHY above)
Results of CSF examination should be provided under Supplementary Information

*☐ ANAESTHESIA/PARAESTHESIA   MIN. HOURS DAYS
Lasting over 24 hours
 Generalized ☐ Localized (indicate site) ☐ _____

*☐ GUILLAIN-BARRÉ SYNDROME   MIN. HOURS DAYS
Progressive subacute weakness of more than one limb (typically symmetrical) with hyporeflexia/areflexia

*☐ PARALYSIS (Do not code if Guillain-Barré Syndrome is coded)   MIN. HOURS DAYS
 Limb paralysis ☐ Facial or cranial paralysis ☐
 Describe _____

*☐ THROMBOCYTOPENIA   MIN. HOURS DAYS
Give lab results under Supplementary Information

☐ OTHER SEVERE OR UNUSUAL EVENTS   MIN. HOURS DAYS
Include any adverse event believed to be related to immunization, that does not fit any of the categories listed above and for which no other cause is clearly established
Report events of clinical interest which require medical attention, and particularly events that are (i) fatal, (ii) life-threatening, (iii) require hospitalization, or (iv) result in residual disability
 DESCRIPTION
 _____
 _____
 _____
 _____

REPORTER'S NAME	TELEPHONE NUMBER ( )	ADDRESS (Institution/No., Street, etc.)		
PROFESSIONAL STATUS: MD ☐ RN ☐ OTHER _____				
SIGNATURE	DATE Year Month Day	City	Province	Postal Code

OUTCOME OF EVENT(S) AT TIME OF REPORT PLEASE FORWARD ANY FOLLOW UP INFORMATION	FULLY RECOVERED ☐	RESIDUAL EFFECTS ☐ (describe)	FATAL ☐	LOST TO ☐ FOLLOW-UP	PENDING ☐

SOUGHT MEDICAL ATTENTION (Emergency room, clinic, family physician etc.) NO ☐ YES ☐ (If yes, include relevant details of treatment under **Supplementary Information**)

HOSPITALIZED BECAUSE OF EVENT(S) NO ☐ YES ☐	LENGTH OF STAY (DAYS) [ ]	DATE ADMITTED	Year	Month	Day

CONCOMITANT MEDICATIONS (exclude those used to treat the adverse event) DRUG(S) GIVEN	MEDICAL HISTORY Please provide information on relevant medical history or concurrent illness (See detailed instructions on reverse)

SUPPLEMENTARY INFORMATION

INSTRUCTIONS FOR COMPLETING REPORT OF A VACCINE-ASSOCIATED ADVERSE EVENT

1. Please use dark ink when completing form to improve legibility of copies.
2. Report only events which have a temporal association with a vaccine and which cannot be attributed to co-existing conditions. **A causal relationship does not need to be proven, and submitting a report does not imply causality.**
3. Events marked with an asterisk (*) must be diagnosed by a physician. Supply relevant details in the SUPPLEMENTARY INFORMATION box.
4. Record interval between vaccine administration and onset of each event in minutes, hours or days.
5. Provide relevant information, when appropriate, in the SUPPLEMENTARY INFORMATION box. Includes details of events diagnosed by physician (see 3 above), results of diagnostic or laboratory tests, hospital treatment, and discharge diagnoses where a vaccinee is hospitalised because of a vaccine-associated adverse event. If appropriate, and preferred, photocopies of original records may be submitted.
6. Provide details of medical history that are relevant to the adverse event(s) reported. Examples include a history of allergies in vaccinee, previous adverse event(s), and concurrent illnesses which may be associated with the current adverse

TO BE COMPLETED BY MEDICAL HEALTH OFFICER RECOMMENDATIONS FOR FURTHER IMMUNIZATION					
	SIGNATURE		DATE	Year	Month	Day
NAME: _____						

202

APPENDIX III
VACCINE PRODUCTS LICENSED IN CANADA

The following list of immunizing agents and the companies licensed to manufacture and/or market them in Canada reflects the situation in 1997 and early 1998, and is not meant to be exhaustive. Products are listed here if they are mentioned in the guide or are related to preventive or therapeutic interventions described in the guide. Some products that are for specialized use or available only under a special access program may not be listed. In addition, new vaccine development has increased in the past few years and the number of products being licensed, sometimes replacing other products, makes it difficult to keep a table such as this one completely up to date. Further, not all licensed products of all manufacturers will necessarily be available in all parts of Canada at all times.

Readers should consult other sources, such as the Compendium of Pharmaceuticals and Specialties (the CPS), their local public health authorities or manufacturers for the latest information about product availability and accessibility. Also, the names used in this table are those in common use and may not be identical with the names used in pharmaceutical compendia.

For new products developed but not yet licensed, or not approved in Canada, that are needed to treat patients in exceptional circumstances, practitioners should contact the Special Access Program of the Therapeutic Products Directorate of Health Canada who have a mandate to authorize the sale of such products. Practitioners should contact the program at 613-941-2108 (after hours 613-941-3061) to initiate a request.

Active Immunizing Agents

Antigen	Descriptive/ brand name	Company	Description or comments
Adenovirus Vaccine		Wyeth-Ayerst Canada Inc.	Type 4, Live Type 7, Live, Oral
BCG Vaccine		Connaught	Intracutaneous (live)
		Biochem Vaccines	Intradermal (live)
Cholera Vaccine		Connaught	Killed, injectable
	MUTACOL BERNA Vaccine	Swiss Serum & Vaccine Institute	Oral, live
Diphtheria Toxoid		Connaught	Fluid D50 Lf/mL Fluid D4, Lf/mL, for immunization of reactors Fluid D0.2 Lf/mL for reaction test
Diphtheria and Tetanus Toxoid (DT, Td and D2T5)	Pediatric Use	Connaught	Adsorbed D25 T5Lf/0.5mL (DT)
		Wyeth-Ayerst Canada Inc.	Adsorbed D12.5 T5Lf/0.5mL
	Adult Use	Connaught	Adsorbed D2 T5Lf/0.5mL (Td for persons > 7 years and recall doses)
		Biochem Vaccines	Adsorbed D2T5Lf/0.5mL (for persons > 7 years and recall doses)
		Wyeth-Ayerst Canada Inc.	Adsorbed D2 T5Lf/0.5mL

Antigen	Descriptive/ brand name	Company	Description or comments
Diphtheria, Pertussis and Tetanus Vaccine (DPT) with Whole-Cell Pertussis Vaccine		Connaught	Adsorbed D25 T5Lf/0.5 mL
	TRI-IMMUNOL	Wyeth-Ayerst Canada Inc.	D12.5T5Lf/0.5 mL
Diphtheria, Tetanus Polio DT-Polio and Td-Polio Vaccine	Td-Polio for 7 years & older	Connaught	Adsorbed D2 T5Lf/0.5 mL
	DT-Polio for children	Connaught	Adsorbed D25 T5Lf/0.5 mL
Diphtheria, Pertussis, Tetanus and Polio Vaccine (DPT-Polio) with Whole-Cell Pertussis		Connaught	Adsorbed D25 T5Lf/0.5 mL
Diphtheria, Pertussis, Tetanus and *Haemophilus influenza* type b Conjugate Vaccine (Diphtheria Toxoid Conjugate) (DPT-Hib)	DPT-Hib	Connaught	Between 18 and 59 months
Diphtheria, Tetanus Toxoid, Pertussis Vaccine (Acellular)	TRIPACEL	Connaught	For primary series and 4th and 5th doses
	ACEL-IMMUNE	Wyeth-Ayerst Canada Inc.	
	INFANRIX	SmithKline Beecham	
Diphtheria, Tetanus Toxoid, Pertussis Vaccine (Acellular) and Polio Vaccine (DTaP-IPV)	QUADRACEL	Connaught	

Antigen	Descriptive/ brand name	Company	Description or comments
Diphtheria & Tetanus Toxoids & Inactivated Poliomyelitis Vaccines combined with *Haemophilus influenzae* type b Conjugate Vaccine (Tetanus Toxoid Conjugate)	PENTA	Connaught	Hib vaccine packaged separately from DPT-Polio, reconstituted prior to administration
Diphtheria & Tetanus Toxoids & Pertussis Vaccine Adsorbed & *Haemophilus influenzae* type b Conjugate Vaccine	TETRAMUNE	Wyeth -Ayerst Canada Inc.	Liquid combination, with whole-cell pertussis vaccine
Haemophilus influenzae type b Conjugate Vaccine (Diphtheria CRM 197 Protein Conjugate)	HibTITER	Wyeth -Ayerst Canada Inc.	Between 2 and 59 months
Haemophilus influenzae type b Conjugate Vaccine (Meningococcal Protein Conjugate)	PedvaxHIB	Merck Frosst Canada Inc.	Between 2 and 59 months
Haemophilus influenzae type b Conjugate Vaccine (Tetanus Toxoid Conjugate)	Act-HIB	Connaught	Between 2 and 59 months
			Active immunizing agent
	PENTACEL	Connaught	Active immunizing agent (reconstituted with Quadracel)

Antigen	Descriptive/ brand name	Company	Description or comments
Hepatitis A Inactivated Vaccine	HAVRIX 1440	SmithKline Beecham	
	HAVRIX 720	SmithKline Beecham	1 year up to and including 18 years of age
Hepatitis A Purified Inactivated Vaccine	VAQTA	Merck Frosst Canada Inc.	Suspension for injection
Hepatitis B Vaccine (Recombinant)	RECOMBIVAX HB	Merck Frosst	
	ENGERIX-B	SmithKline Beecham Pharma	
Hep A, Heb B	TWINRIX	SmithKline Beecham Pharma	For adults
	TWINRIX JUNIOR		For children
Influenza Vaccine	FLUZONE	Connaught	Whole virus, Split virus
	VAXIGRIP	Connaught	Split virus
	FLUVIRAL	Biochem Vaccines	Whole virus, Split virus
	FLUARIX	SmithKline Beecham Pharma	Split virus
Japanese Encephalitis Virus Vaccine	JE-VAX	Biken	Inactivated
	JE-VAX	Connaught	Inactivated
Measles Vaccine		Connaught	Live, attenuated
	RIMEVAX	Biochem Vaccines	Live, attenuated
Measles and Rubella Virus Vaccine	MoRu-VIRATEN BERNA VACCINE	Swiss Serum & Vaccine Institute	Live, attenuated
	EOLARIX	SmithKline Beecham Pharma	
	RUDI-ROUVAX	Connaught	
Measles, Mumps and Rubella Vaccine	MMR II	Merck Frosst Canada Inc.	Single dose vials

Antigen	Descriptive/ brand name	Company	Description or comments
Meningococcal Polysaccharide Vaccine	Meningococcal Polysaccharide Vaccine	Connaught	Groups A and C
			Groups A, C, Y and W-135
	MENCEVAX AC	SmithKline Beecham Pharma	Groups A and C
Mumps Skin Test Antigen		Connaught	
Mumps Vaccine	MUMPSVAX	Merck Frosst Canada Inc.	Live, attenuated
Pertussis Vaccine, monovalent	Whole cell	Connaught	
	Acel-P (acellular)	Wyeth-Ayerst Canada Inc.	Adsorbed
Pneumococcal Vaccine	PNEUMOVAX 23	Merck Frosst Canada Inc.	Polyvalent: 23 capsular types
	PNU-IMUNE 23	Wyeth-Ayerst Canada Inc.	
	PNEUMO 23	Connaught	
Poliovirus Vaccine	OPV	Connaught	Live, oral (Sabin) trivalent
Poliomyelitis Vaccine (IPV)	IMOVAX Polio	Connaught	Inactivated (Salk) trivalent: vero cell origin
		Connaught	Inactivated (Salk) trivalent: MRC5
Rabies Vaccine		Connaught	Inactivated Human Diploid Cell
Rubella Vaccine		Connaught	Live, attenuated
		Biochem Vaccines	Live, attenuated

Antigen	Descriptive/ brand name	Company	Description or comments
Tetanus Toxoid		Connaught	Fluid T10Lf/mL
			Adsorbed T5Lf/0.5mL
		Biochem Vaccines	Adsorbed T5Lf/0.5mL
		Wyeth-Ayerst Canada Inc.	
Tetanus and Polio Vaccine		Connaught	Adsorbed T5Lf/0.5mL
Tuberculin	TUBERSOL (MANTOUX)	Connaught	
	Tuberculin Old Tine Test	Wyeth-Ayerst Canada Inc.	
	PPD-B (Mantoux)	Connaught	
Typhoid Vaccine	TYPHIM VI VACCINE	Connaught	*Salmonella typhi* Vi capsular polysaccharide
	VIVOTIF BERNA VACCINE	Swiss Serum & Vaccine Institute	Live, oral, capsular, for persons $\geq$ 6 years of age
	VIVOTIF L BERNA VACCINE	Swiss Serum & Vaccine Institute	Liquid, for persons $\geq$ 3 years
Yellow Fever Vaccine		Connaught	Live, attenuated

Passive Immunizing Agents

Antigen	Descriptive/ brand name	Company	Description or comments
Botulism Anti-toxin (Equine)		Connaught	Type E
		Connaught	Type A, B and E
Diptheria antitoxin (Equine)		Connaught	
Hepatitis B Immune Globulin	BAYHEP	Bayer	Solvent detergent treated
	H-BIG	Alpha Therapeutic Corp.	
Tetanus Immune Globulin	TETABULLIN	Österreichische Institut Für Haemoderivate	
	BAYTET	Bayer	Solvent detergent treated
Varicella - Zoster Immune Globulin		Massachusetts P.H. Biologics Laboratories	Human Origin
Respiratory Syncytial Virus Immune Globulin	RESPIGAM	MedImmune Inc	
Immune Globulin (human)	GAMMABULIN	Österreichische Institut Für Haemoderivate	
	BAYGAM	Bayer	Solvent detergent treated
Immune Globulin, Intravenous (human)	GAMIMUNE	Bayer	Solvent detergent treated 5% and 10%
	GAMMAGARD S/D	Baxter	Solvent detergent treated 5%
	IVEEGAM	Österreichische Institut Für Haemoderivate	5%

Appendix IV
LICENSED MANUFACTURERS OR DISTRIBUTORS (contacts for vaccines distributed in Canada)

Connaught Laboratories Limited
c/o Pasteur Mérieux Connaught Canada
1755 Steeles Avenue West
North York, Ontario M2R 3T4
Tel: 1-888-621-1146

The Research Foundation for Microbial
  Diseases of Osaka University (BIKEN)
3-1 Yamada-oka
Suita, Osaka
565 Japan
Tel: 011-81-6-875-25-4171

SmithKline Beecham Pharma Inc.
2030 Bristol Circle
Oakville, Ontario L6H 5V2
Tel: 1-800-567-1550

Merck Frosst Canada Inc.
P.O. Box 1005
Pointe-Claire-Dorval
Quebec H9R 4P8
Tel: (514) 428-2642

Wyeth-Ayerst Canada Inc.
110 Sheppard Avenue East
North York, Ontario M2N 6R5
Tel: (416) 226-7612

Swiss Serum and Vaccine Institute
c/o Berna Products Corp
1555 Bonhill, Unit 2
Mississauga, Ontario L5T 1Y5
Tel: 1-800-533-5899

Biochem Vaccines Inc.
2323 Parc Technologique Blvd.
Sainte-Foy, Quebec G1P 4R8
Tel: (418) 650-0010

Massachusetts Public Health
  Biologic Laboratories
c/o MedImmune Inc.
35 West Watkins Mill Road
Gaithersburg, MD 20878
Tel: (800) 959-1427

Bayer, Inc.
77 Belfield Road,
Etobicoke, Ontario M9W 1G6
Tel: 1-800-268-1331

Baxter Corporation
4 Robert Speck Parkway, Suite 700
Mississauga, Ontario L4E 3Y4
Tel: 1-800-387-8399

Alpha Therapeutic Corporation
5555 Valley Blvd
Los Angeles, CA 90032
Tel: (213) 225-2221

Osterreichisches Institut
  Für Haemoderivate
c/o Immuno (Canada) Ltd.
6635 Kitimat Road, Suite 30
Mississauga, Ontario L5N 6J2
Tel: (905) 858-3539

Cangene, Inc.
104 Chancellor Metheson Road
Winnipeg, Manitoba R3T 5Y3
Tel: (204) 989-6850

INDEX

Canadian Immunization Guide
— Fifth Edition

Additional copies available from
the Canadian Medical Association

Please send me _____ copies of the *Canadian Immunization Guide* today!

Price: $10.95 in Canada; elsewhere US$10.95

Please add $3 shipping and handling. In Canada, add 7% GST/HST.

All orders must be prepaid.

Bulk order discounts available. Contact CMA Member Service Centre for details.

Language: ❏ English ❏ French

❏ Enclosed cheque or money order (payable to the Canadian Medical Association)

❏ Credit card ❏ VISA ❏ MasterCard ❏ American Express

Card number .... Expiry date ....

Name ....

Address ....

City .... Province ....

Postal code .... Telephone (.........) ....

Email address ....

Signature .... Total $ ....

Mail to
Member Service Centre
Canadian Medical Association
1867 Alta Vista Dr.
Ottawa ON K1G 3Y6

Credit card payments may be made
toll free: 888 855-2555
phone: 613 731-8610 x2307
fax: 613 731-9102
email: cmamsc@cma.ca

GST registration number 121 765 705